$CCC = 300$

$CD = 400$

$CDXLIX = \text{449}$

$CM = 900.$

$I - 1$

$\frac{1}{13}$    $| V | - 5$   $L50$

$\downarrow$    $X - 10$

$X\frac{1}{3}$    $L - 50$

      $\frac{-33\frac{1}{3}}{33,00}$

$1 = 100\%$   $C - 100$

$D = 500$

$M = 1000.$

     $\begin{array}{r} .1256 \\ 100 \\ \hline 12.56\% \end{array}$

     $\begin{array}{c} 1000 \ 900 \ 70 \ 7 \\ M \ | \ CM \ | \ L \ x \ x \ V \ I \ I \end{array}$

$1977 = M \ C M \ L \ x \ x \ V \ I \ I$

     $\frac{1}{3} = 3\overline{)1.00} \; .3$

$\frac{1}{2} = 50\%$

$\frac{1}{2}\% = \frac{1}{2}\% \text{ of } 1\%.$

$\frac{1}{5} \ \frac{\cancel{4945}\ 9}{}$

$\frac{1}{3} \ \frac{15-}{45}$

$\frac{1}{9} \ \frac{5-}{45}$

gal = 4

pt, O = pint

$q^t$ = quarter

$m_{\cancel{4}}$

cc

L

K

mg.

$\frac{1}{\cancel{3}}$ = gram

$\cancel{3}$ ounce.

1 cl · m = 1 gram

T = table spoon 15 cc

t = teaspoon. 4 cc

$7\frac{1}{2} = \frac{7\ \overline{ss}}{VIISS}$

$\overline{ss} = \frac{1}{2}$ one half.

# DRUGS

*Third Edition*

# &

# SOLUTIONS

## A Programed Introduction

CLAIRE B. KEANE, R.N., B.S., M. Ed.

and

SYBIL M. FLETCHER, R.N.

1975   W. B. SAUNDERS COMPANY   Philadelphia • London • Toronto

W. B. Saunders Company:    West Washington Square
                           Philadelphia, PA  19105

                           12 Dyott Street
                           London, WC1A  1DB

                           833 Oxford Street
                           Toronto, Ontario M8Z  5T9, Canada

**Library of Congress Cataloging in Publication Data**

Keane, Claire Brackman.
    Drugs and solutions.

    1. Pharmaceutical arithmetic–Programmed instruction.
I. Fletcher, Sybil M., joint author. II. Title: [DNLM:
1. Mathematics–Programmed instruction. 2. Pharmacy–Programmed
instruction. QV16 K24d]

RS57.K4 1975   615′ .4′01513   74–21014

ISBN 0–7216–5342–1

Drugs and Solutions                          ISBN  0–7216–5342–1

Last digit is the print number:   9  8  7  6  5  4  3  2  1

# INTRODUCTION

The material in this textbook is programed. If you have never used a programed text before, you will be in for a few surprises when you settle down to the business of using this one to learn about the dosages of drugs and solutions.

First, you will have to use this text—not just read it. You must actively participate in the programed exercises we have written for you. In fact, this is the chief purpose of any programed text: the active participation of the learner.

Second, we hope that you will accept this material in the spirit in which it was written, that is, that learning can be both exciting and rewarding when we are truly interested in achieving the goals we have set for ourselves, and when we are willing to put forth the effort necessary to reach these goals.

The content of this programed text is divided into short, logically organized units called *frames.* Each frame asks you a question, and this is where your participation comes in. You must try to answer each question as best you can before moving on to the next one. If you have read the frame carefully (and if we have written it clearly!), you should have no trouble in answering the question. The correct answer for each frame appears in a special column beside the question frame. Each frame is numbered, and the same number identifies its answer. Tear off the perforated "slider" attached to the back cover of the book and use it to mask the printed answers until you have written out your own. You can write your answers either in the blank spaces in the program itself or on a separate sheet of paper. Whichever method you use, however, it is most important that you actually *write* your answers and not just "think" them.

Since we have given you the correct answers to every question, we obviously are not trying to trick you or test you. You will receive the greatest benefit from this program by being entirely honest with yourself and by freely recognizing when you don't understand something and have written a wrong answer. You can then go on to the special frames we have written for those who don't get the correct answer on the first try.

For a little practice, try these two frames:

**A**

question

**A**

Programed instruction gives the student information in short, easy-to-read steps. The learner reads the information and then answers a question about it. In each frame, the reader is asked to make an active response by answering a

_____ .

*B*

**B**

Each person is an individual who learns in a unique way and at her own rate of speed. Some learn more rapidly than others, and some can recall things they have learned in the past more efficiently than others. The material in this text is presented so that some students can skip over material that they already know.

Each student using this program can progress at her own individual rate of
speed _____.

That was easy, wasn't it? In fact, you may have found it too *simple,* but don't become complacent. We expect you to *think* as you read each frame of the text. Then, at the end of each Part, we will give you a review test, so that you can be sure that you thoroughly understand the information you have been given. Accept each question as a challenge to you as an intelligent, thinking person—the only kind of person who can make a real contribution to health care.

# A NOTE TO THE INSTRUCTOR

One of the greatest challenges in writing programed instruction is that it requires the writer to establish a clear, precise picture of what is expected of the learner. Before we undertook this program, we wrote the objectives that follow for the learner. We encourage you as an instructor to read the objectives and to make them clear to your students, so that they will understand specifically what is to be accomplished by using this text.

This text should not be used as one would use a conventional textbook. Programed instruction is designed primarily for *self-instruction.* Each student should be allowed to work independently at his own pace. The function of the instructor is to provide help in areas in which the student may have difficulty or to supplement the material with information pertinent to what the student is expected to learn.

In this third edition we have added three new sections: pediatric dosages, regulation of the flow of intravenous fluids, and conversion of Fahrenheit and Celsius temperatures. The latter two sections, while not directly related to the administration of medications and pre-paration of solutions, do involve some arithmetical skills. They are included in answer to requests from instructors who are familiar with the first two editions of this book. Additional clinical situations have been provided in many units and practice problems are given at the end of the text.

The many helpful suggestions and criticisms received from our readers are appreciated. We hope that changes, additions, and deletions made in this edition will improve its effectiveness and increase its value to students and instructors.

# A STATEMENT OF OBJECTIVES

1. The learner will be able to name and describe the three systems of measurement used in weighing and measuring drugs and solutions.

2. Given a list of the various symbols and abbreviations used to express units of weight and measure in the three systems, the learner will be able to read these symbols and abbreviations correctly and to interpret them in writing.

3. Provided with a list of specific quantities of medications, the learner will be able to write each of the dosages using proper symbols, abbreviations, and numbers.

4. Given a list of the more commonly used units of weight and measure in the apothecaries', metric, and household systems, the learner will be able to identify the system from which each unit is taken and to give its approximate equivalent in one or more alternate systems of measurements.

5. Presented with situations in which dosage is ordered in one system of measurement and is available only in another system, the learner will be

able to demonstrate a ready knowledge of conversion by calculating the correct amount of drug to be given to the patient.

6. Given situations in which a solution for parenteral administration must be prepared from a powdered drug, the learner will be aware of the necessity for reading the instructions provided by the manufacturer and for following these instructions precisely when adding the proper amount of diluent to obtain the correct dosage.

7. Confronted with situations in which a small amount of solution must be prepared from hypodermic tablets, the learner will be able to determine the number of tablets to be dissolved and the amount of diluent necessary to obtain the correct dosage.

8. Given situations in which the dosage must be calculated from a stock solution, the learner will be able to set up each problem according to ratio and proportion and to determine the correct amount of solution to be given

9. Presented with situations in which the drug ordered is dispensed in units, the learner will be able to calculate the correct dosage to be given from the amount on hand.

10. Given situations in which the dosage of insulin must be administered from a syringe other than an insulin syringe, the learner will be able to determine the number of milliliters or minims that the patient is to receive.

11. Given a situation in which the rate of flow for continuous administration of intravenous fluids

must be calculated, the learner will be able to determine the number of drops to be administered per minute.

12. Given situations in which a large amount of solution must be prepared from a pure drug, the learner will be able to set up a proportion for the purpose of determining the amount of pure drug to be dissolved in a given amount of diluent to achieve the correct concentration in each instance.

13. Provided with theoretical situations in which a large amount of solution must be prepared from a stock solution, the learner will be able to set up a proportion for each situation and to determine the amount of stock solution to be added to a given amount of diluent to achieve the correct strength in each instance.

14. Given a situation in which the dosage of a drug for a pediatric patient is prescribed in dosage per kilogram of body weight, the learner will be able to convert pound to kilogram in order to give the correct dosage.

15. Given a situation in which there is no reference book available as a guide to pediatric dosage, the learner will be able to use Clark's rule to estimate the average pediatric dosage for certain medications.

16. The learner will be able to calculate approximate equivalents between Celsius (centigrade) and Fahrenheit temperatures.

# CONTENTS

# PART ONE

# INTRODUCTION TO SYSTEMS OF MEASUREMENT

**1**

**1**

In the early history of drug preparation, medicines were administered in the form of powders or brews made from herbs, roots, and other parts of plants. There was no way of knowing exactly *how much* medication a patient was receiving, because no standards had been set for accurately weighing and measuring drugs.

Today, when a physician prescribes a drug, he is assured of the accuracy of the dosage because there are universally accepted standards or systems for the measurement of drugs.

**2**

system
measurement

**2**

A universally accepted standard which assures accuracy in the weighing and measuring of drugs is called a _____ _____ of _____.

**3**

apothecaries'

**3**

In the United States we now use two systems of measurement in preparing and administering drugs. Of the two, the *apothecaries'* system is the older. It was brought to the United States from England during the colonial period.

A system of measurement brought to the United States in the eighteenth century, and still used today in the preparation and administration of drugs, is the _____ system.

**4**

metric

**4**

Another system by which drugs are weighed and measured is the metric system. This system is more convenient than the apothecaries' system, and it is the one used in the official listings of drugs.

Since most drugs are prepared and dispensed from an official listing, the system most frequently used in the weighing and measuring of drugs is the _____ system.

**5**

apothecaries'
    metric (either)
    order)

**5**

Two systems used for weighing and measuring drugs in the United States are the _____ system and the _____ system.

**6**

**6**

The administration of drugs would be much simpler if all drugs were prescribed, weighed, measured, and dispensed according to one universal system of measurement. However, even though the apothecaries' system is gradually being replaced by the metric system, each system is in current use, and you should be familiar with both.

Sometimes a physician will prescribe a dosage of a drug using the apothecaries'

apothecaries'
metric

system, when the drug is dispensed according to the units of the metric system. When this happens, you must be able to translate, or convert, from units of measure in the _____ system to units of measure in the _____ system.

**7**

household

**7**

Drugs such as milk of magnesia, cough syrup and other medications sold in drug stores and administered in the home as well as in the hospital are usually measured and administered in a household article such as a teaspoon or a tablespoon. Although these articles do not give so completely accurate a measurement as the metric and apothecaries' systems, they are recognized and used as units of measure in the household system.

Another system of measurement used for measuring drugs commonly sold in drug stores and taken in the home is the _____ system.

# Post-Test on Systems of Measurement

A. **Write the correct word or words to complete each of the following statements:**

1. A universally accepted standard which assures accuracy in weighing and measuring drugs is called a _____ of measurement.

2. The two principal systems used for weighing and measuring drugs in the United States are the_____ system and the_____system.

3. A system of measurement which is not completely accurate but is sometimes used for administering medications in the home is the_____ system.

4. The system of measurement used most often in preparing and dispensing drugs is the _____ system.

5. An older system of measurement that is frequently used by physicians in prescribing drugs is the_____ system.

# PART TWO

# THE APOTHECARIES' SYSTEM

# UNIT I

# Units of Measure in the Apothecaries' System

**1**

units
measure

**1**

Before we can understand any system of measurement, we must have some concept of the *units* of measure in that system. For example, inches, feet, and yards are units of linear measure.

When you administer drugs prescribed in the apothecaries' system, you must be familiar with the_____of _____in that system.

**2**

apothecaries'

**2**

Americans are familiar with many of the units of measure in the apothecaries' system because we use them in our everyday life. We buy gasoline by the gallon, milk by the quart, and cream by the pint. The gallon, the quart, and the pint are all units of measure in the _____ system.

**3**

12 irrigations

**3**

Now try this problem: You must prepare 3 gallons of Zephiran solution for vaginal irrigations. If each irrigation requires 1 quart of Zephiran solution, then 3 gallons of the solution would be sufficient for _____ irrigations.

If your answer was correct, please go on to Frame 6. If you did not get the correct answer or are not sure how the answer was obtained go to Frame 4.

**4**

12 irrigations

**4**

Perhaps you don't know the apothecaries' system as well as we thought. There are 4 quarts in 1 gallon. Three gallons of solution would be sufficient for 3 × 4 or _____ irrigations.

**5**

2 one-gallon jugs

**5**

Now see if you can get this one. If we needed to prepare 8 quarts of a sterile solution in one-gallon containers, it would be necessary to sterilize • 2 one-gallon jugs/4 one-gallon jugs • before preparing the solution.

**6**

2 quarts

**6**

Let us suppose that you must prepare enough saline solution for 4 irrigations during the day. If you will need 1 pint of saline solution for each irrigation, you should prepare • 1 quart/2 quarts • of the solution. If your answer came out 1 quart, please go on to Frame 7; if it was 2 quarts, go on to Frame 8.

**7**

**7**

You must have forgotten that 2 pints are equal to 1 quart. If there are 2 pints in 1

**2 quarts**

quart, then 4 pints would be equal to
_____ quart(s).

---

**8**

quart
pint
ounce (or fluid
    ounce)

**8**

The next smaller unit in the apothecaries' system, after the pint, is the *fluid*
ounce. Most people are familiar with the
word ounce used in relation to the
weighing of solids; however, the nurse
will most often see ounce used in measuring liquid drugs. The measurement
may be written as ounce or *fluid* ounce.
Either term is correct.

In descending order of size, the units of
the apothecaries' system for measuring
liquids are: the gallon, the_____,
the_____, and the _____.

---

**9**

quart
gallon


1 quart

**9**

You now know four units of measure in
the apothecaries' system: the ounce, the
pint, the_____ , and the_____.

There are 32 ounces in 1 quart. If an
infant is receiving 4 ounces of formula
per feeding, you would need to prepare
_____ quart(s) of formula for 8
feedings.

---

**10**

4 1/2 quarts

**10**

If a child drinks 6 eight-ounce glasses of
milk each day, you will need_____
quart(s) for a three-day supply.

If you answered this correctly, go on to Frame 13. If you don't see how we got this figure, go on to Frame 11.

## 11

4 1/2 quarts

## 11

There are two steps in this problem. First, you must determine the total number of ounces the child will drink in *one* day (6 × 8 ounces = (equal) 48 ounces). A three-day supply would be 3 × 48 ounces, or 144 ounces. To change ounces to quarts, you would divide this number by 32 (because there are 32 ounces in a quart). Therefore your answer is _____ quart(s).

## 12

2 1/4 quarts

## 12

A physician orders milk and cream for a patient with a peptic ulcer. The dosage is 3 ounces every hour. If you were responsible for ordering the milk and cream every morning, you would order _____ quart(s) of the mixture for a 24-hour period.

## 13

1 1/2 quarts

## 13

Suppose that you are caring for a patient who receives 4 ounces of tube feeding every 2 hours. Since the tube feeding is prepared in quarts and is ordered only once a day, you would order _____ quart(s) for a 24-hour period.

1 pint

Weak and debilitated patients sometimes receive dietary supplements to increase their intake of food elements. If a physician orders 4 ounces to be given 4 times a day, you would need _____ pint(s) for a one-day supply.

dram

When we measure liquids we usually choose the unit of measure that most nearly represents the amount we need. Thus, if we need large amounts, we measure the liquid in quarts rather than ounces: and if we need smaller amounts, we use ounces rather than quarts. Should we need to measure an even smaller amount, we could use drams.

In the apothecaries' system, a unit of measure that is smaller than the ounce is the _____ .

The standard medicine glass used in many hospitals for the administration of

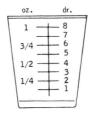

liquid medication by mouth is a one-ounce glass. This small glass is usually marked, or graduated, in drams. Sometimes the glass is graduated in ounces, drams, and other units.

8 drams

In the drawing, you can see that 1 ounce is equal to _____ dram(s).

**17**

**17**

4 drams

If a physician orders 1/2 ounce of medication for a patient, you would give the patient _____ dram(s).

**18**

**18**

16 drams

Sometimes a physician will order 2 ounces of a certain medication. This is equal to approximately _____ dram(s).

**19**

**19**

minim

Another unit of measure in the apothecaries' system is the *minim.* The word *minim* means "the least."

The smallest unit of liquid measure in the apothecaries' system is the _____.

**20**

**20**

minims

When a minim is used as a unit of measure, it is usually because the drug to be administered is very potent. When such a drug is to be given by injection, prepare it in a syringe graduated in _____ .

**21**

Most textbooks on drugs and solutions contain a number of tables of equivalents. It is not necessary for you to memorize all of these tables, because you already know some equivalents of liquid measure in the apothecaries' system from working the previous problems.

How many equivalents do you already know in the following table?

Fluid measure in the apothecaries' system

| | | |
|---|---|---|
| 4 quarts | ———— quarts = | 1 gallon |
| 2 pints | ———— pints = | 1 quart |
| 32 ounces | ———— ounces = | 1 quart |
| 8 drams | ———— drams = | 1 ounce |

**22**

solid

**22**

All the units in the table in Frame 21 pertained to liquid measure. There is, however, one unit of weight in the apothecaries' system that is still used quite frequently for solid drugs, and it should be included here. This unit of weight originally was compared to a grain of wheat, and is very conveniently called a grain.

In the apothecaries' system the quart, the ounce, and the dram are three units used in measuring liquids; the grain is a unit sometimes used in weighing ———————— drugs.

grain

Although there are many other units of weight in the apothecaries' system, the grain is the only one that you are likely to use.

Since all the other units have become generally obsolete, the only unit of weight in the apothecaries' system that we will be concerned with here is the
_____ .

## UNIT II

# Abbreviations, Symbols, and Numbers in the Apothecaries' System

*1*

**1**

You have probably been in the health field long enough to realize that health personnel speak and write a language all their own. You have struggled through Latin prefixes and suffixes, trying to make some sense out of medical terminology—but brace yourself, there is more to come! There are also a number of abbreviations and symbols that you must know before you can give medications to your patients.

**2**

gallon . . . . . .gal.
quart . . . . . .qt.
pint . . . . . .pt.
ounce . . . . . .oz.

**2**

Don't get discouraged! Things really aren't as bad as we have suggested. You are already familiar with some of the abbreviations used for units of measure in the apothecaries' system. Look at the list below and see how well you can do:

| Unit of measure | Abbreviation |
|---|---|
| gallon | _____ |
| quart | _____ |
| pint | _____ |
| ounce | _____ |

If you missed any of the abbreviations in Frame 2, go back and study them carefully. We will use these abbreviations often in the frames to come.

**3**

gr.

**3**

The abbreviations for dram and grain are easy. We just use the first two letters of the word and then put a period at the end. Therefore, the abbreviation for dram is dr., and the abbreviation for grain is _____ .

**4**

the symbol

**4**

In the preceding frames we learned a few abbreviations, but we did not say anything about symbols. Symbols are letters or signs that are used as substitutes for an entire word. The sign ℥ is · the symbol/ an abbreviation · for ounce.

**5**

℥

**5**

The symbol for ounce is ℥. The symbol for dram is ʒ. Because they are so similar, it is important to avoid confusing the two. In charting medications on a patient's medical record, you should use the symbol · ʒ / ℥ · to designate ounce.

**6**

ʒ

**6**

If a physician orders a medication in drams, you would use the symbol _____ in charting the medication.

**7**

minims

**7**

The symbol for minim is easy to remember because it resembles a small m. It is written like this: ℞. If you saw a syringe marked with the symbol ℞, you would know that it was calibrated in_____.

**8**

Roman numerals

**8**

You remember that we have called the apothecaries' system a very old system of measurement. You also know that Roman numerals have been used for counting since ancient times. It would be fairly safe, then, to guess that the numbers used to designate amounts in the apothecaries' system would be_____

_____ .

**9**

**9**

Reading Roman numerals should be nothing new to you. They are used in chapter headings, on clocks and sundials, and in many other places. Since you will be using small Roman numerals in reading prescriptions and charting dosages of drugs, test yourself on the following:

| | Roman numeral | Arabic number |
|---|---|---|
| 1 | i | _____ |
| 4 | iv | _____ |
| 5 | v | _____ |
| 7 | vii | _____ |
| 9 | ix | _____ |
| 10 | x | _____ |
| 22 | xxii | _____ |
| 34 | xxxiv | _____ |

If you missed any of the small Roman numerals in Frame 9, you should go on to Frame 10 and review them. If all your answers were right, go on to Frame 18.

## *10*

xv

## 10

We are going to consider only the Roman numerals that designate the smaller amounts, because these are the only ones that you will use in reading physician's orders and charting medications. The two most important numerals to remember are x and v. The x represents 10 and the v represents 5. If we combine x and v, we get 15. The Roman numeral for 15 is _____ .

**11**

added to

**11**

We can see that by writing v to the right of x we have added v, which is 5, to x, which is 10. When a numeral follows one of larger value, it is · added to / subtracted from · the numeral it follows.

**12**

three

**12**

The smaller Roman numerals other than x and v are easy to read. The i is one, ii is two and iii is _____ .

**13**

13

**13**

If the smaller numerals to the right are always added to the numeral of larger value, then xiii is the same as the Arabic number_____ .

**14**

9

**14**

We have seen that the position of one Roman numeral in relation to another is very important. Whenever a smaller numeral follows one of larger value, the numerals are added. But if a smaller numeral precedes one of larger value, it is subtracted from the large numeral. Therefore, ix means 10 minus 1, or _____ .

**15**

4

**15**

You know that i is less than v. The Roman numeral iv, therefore, represents the Arabic number _____ .

**16**

30

**16**

Sometimes we see a combination of Roman numerals that are of equal value; for example, xxx. When the numerals are written this way, all their values are added. Thus, xxx equals 10+10+10, or

_____ .

**17**

8
16
24
35
14

**17**

Let's go through another set of Roman numerals and their Arabic equivalents, to be sure you understand them thoroughly:

| Roman numeral | Arabic number |
|---------------|---------------|
| viii | _____ |
| xvi | _____ |
| xxiv | _____ |
| xxxv | _____ |
| xiv | _____ |

**18**

ss.

**18**

To express parts of a unit in the apothecaries' system, we use common fractions such as 2/3 or 3/4. The only exception to this rule is 1/2, which is expressed by the Latin abbreviation ss.

When we wish to express the fraction 1/2 in the apothecaries' system, we use the abbreviation _____ .

**19**

℥ ii

**19**

There is one more thing you should know about writing weights and measures in the apothecaries' system. That is, that the numbers indicating the amount to be given are always written *after* the symbol or abbreviation for the unit of measure. If you were charting 2 ounces of a medication, you would write it as _____. (Be sure to use the symbol for ounce.)

**20**

2 1/2 ounces

**20**

Now you should be ready to read and write any unit of measure in the apothecaries' system according to the rules you have learned.

Let's say that a physician orders milk of magnesia ℥ iss. This should be read as

_____.

**21**

1 1/2 ounces

**21**

If a physician orders mineral oil ℥ iss., you would give the patient _____ _____of the drug.

**22**

4 ounces

**22**

If the medicine card reads ℥ iv, you would pour_____ of the medication.

**23**

℥ iii

**23**

Suppose you were instructed to give 3 ounces of a certain medication. In charting this you would write the symbol and amount as _____ .

**24**

2 drams

**24**

An order reading cascara ℥ ii means that the patient is to receive _____ of cascara.

**25**

℥ i

**25**

If a physician orders 1 dram of Elixir of Donnatal, you would chart the symbol and amount as _____ .

**26**

12 minims

**26**

Suppose that you have an order written: tincture of belladonna ♏ xii. You should read the amount as _____ .

**27**

♏ iv

**27**

If a physician orders 4 minims of a certain drug, you would chart this amount as _____ .

**28**

**28**

Here we run into some difficulty with the apothecaries' system, and can sympathize with those who wish to do away with it. We have said that Roman numerals are used in the apothecaries' system and that parts of a whole are expressed as common fractions. The Romans, however, had no way of expressing fractions such as 1/4 and 1/8 in numbers. In fact, the only common fraction we can indicate in Latin is 1/2, which is abbreviated ss. All other common fractions must be written in Arabic numbers.

gr. 1/4

Therefore, to express 1/4 grain, you would write gr._____.

# UNIT III

# Review of Fractions

*1*

**1**

Inconvenient as the apothecaries' system may be, we are still using it, and you must know fractions and how to use them in calculations if you are going to administer medications intelligently.

The word fraction indicates one or more equal parts of a unit. If a unit is divided into two or more equal parts, the parts of the unit are referred to, and written, as fractions.

**2**

$4 \div 6$

**2**

In the fraction 4/6, the line between the two numbers is read "divided by." You could write 4/6 as _____ ÷ _____.

**3**

**3**

The number below the fraction line indicates the way a unit is divided, and is called the denominator. Look at this drawing:

| | |
|---|---|
| 3<br>3 | Since the unit (the whole circle) has been divided into _____ parts, the denominator of the fraction is _____ . |
| **4**<br><br>smaller | **4**<br><br>We know that the denominator indicates the way a unit is divided, and also that the more we divide a unit the smaller the parts will be. In other words, the larger the denominator, the · smaller/larger · the size of each part. |
| **5**<br><br>smaller | **5**<br><br>The fraction 1/300 represents a · larger/smaller · amount than 1/100. |
| **6**<br><br>less | **6**<br><br>Suppose that you needed to give a patient gr. 1/8 of morphine sulfate, and the only tablets on hand were gr. 1/4 tablets. Is gr. 1/8 more or less than gr. 1/4?_____ . |
| **7** | **7**<br><br>The number above the fraction line is called the numerator, and indicates the number of parts *taken* from the unit. In the drawing, the shaded area indicates the part taken: |

1
3

Here, the numerator is _____ and the denominator is _____.

**8**

(a) proper
(b) improper
(c) mixed
number

**8**

Life would be much simpler for everyone if there were only one kind of fraction. Actually there are three, and examples of each kind are given below. See if you can remember from your earlier experience with arithmetic what these are called, and write down the name of each kind of fraction beside the example given.:

(a) 1/3 _____ fraction
(b) 8/5 _____ fraction
(c) 2 1/4 _____ _____

If you got all three answers to Frame 8 correct, go on to Frame 18. If you aren't sure about these three kinds of fractions, continue with Frame 9.

**9**

**9**

There are three types of fractions: proper fractions, improper fractions, and mixed numbers. When we think of the word "fraction," we think of a unit divided into equal parts. A proper fraction refers to the division of only one unit into two or more equal

parts                    _____ .

---

**10**

number
divided
numerator
denominator

**10**

We have seen that the numerator indicates the _____ of equal parts taken from a unit, and that the denominator indicates the way in which the unit is _____ . In a proper fraction, the _____ cannot be larger than the _____ .

---

**11**

proper

**11**

In a proper fraction, the denominator is always larger than the numerator. Fractions in which the numerator is *smaller* than the denominator are called _____ fractions.

---

**12**

larger

**12**

The opposite of proper is improper. Proper fractions have numerators that are smaller than their denominators. In improper fractions, the numerators are _____ than the denominators.

---

**13**

**13**

Improper fractions indicate the division of more than one unit. In the drawing below, you can see that two units have been divided into fourths. The five parts

5/4

taken have been shaded. We can represent this division by writing the improper fraction _____ .

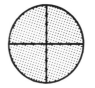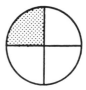

1/4

**14**

If in the drawing in Frame 13 you counted all the shaded areas together, you could say that they represented the improper fraction 5/4. If you counted these shaded areas as parts taken from *two separate* units, you could say that they represented a mixed *number,* 1 and

_____ .

(fraction)

are

**15**

A mixed number represents one or more whole units, plus part of another unit. An improper fraction represents parts of more than one unit. Thus, improper fractions and mixed numbers · are/are not · two different ways of expressing the same amount.

proper
mixed number
improper fraction

**16**

Therefore, 1/2 is a(n) _____ fraction; 1 1/2 is a(n) _____ _____ ; and 6/5 is a(n) _____ _____ .

## 17

### 17

(a) proper
   fraction
(b) mixed
   number
(c) improper
   fraction
(d) mixed
   number
(e) proper
   fraction

There are three types of fractions: proper fractions, improper fractions, and mixed numbers. Look at the following examples and say which type each fraction represents:

(a) 3/8 is a(n) _____
   _____.

(b) 21 3/4 is a(n) _____
   _____.

(c) 9/8 is a(n) _____
   _____.

(d) 2 5/8 is a(n) _____
   _____.

(e) 13/15 is a(n) _____
   _____.

## 18

### 18

improper fraction

Because improper fractions and mixed numbers represent two different ways of expressing the same amount, it really doesn't matter which we use. There are times, however, when it is much easier to work arithmetic problems if we write the mixed number as a(n) _____
_____.

## 19

### 19

15/2

Can you change a mixed number to an improper fraction? The mixed number 7 1/2 may be written as the improper fraction _____ .

If you feel confident in changing mixed

numbers to improper fractions, go on to Frame 25. If you would like a review go to Frame 20.

**20**

1 × 8

**20**

We can change any mixed number to an improper fraction by following two quick and easy steps. First we multiply the whole number by the denominator of the fraction. For instance, to change the mixed number 1 7/8 to an improper fraction, our first step would be to multiply _____ × _____ .

**21**

15

**21**

We have multiplied the whole number 1 by the denominator of the fraction, 8. Now we take the result of this multiplication and add it to the numerator of the fraction. After adding 8 to 7, our answer is _____ eighths.

**22**

40
43

**22**

Let's try both steps together, and change 10 3/4 to an improper fraction.
    *First step:*  10 × 4 = _____ fourths
    *Second step:*  add 3 fourths
    *Your answer* _____ fourths

**23**

**23**

Now suppose you needed to change 12 3/5 to an improper fraction.

$12 \times 5 = 60$
add 3
answer: 63

First: _____ × _____ = _____ fifths
Second: add _____ fifths
Your answer: _____ fifths

**24**

(a) 21/8
(b) 11/8
(c) 20/7
(d) 41/9

**24**

Just for practice, change these mixed numbers to improper fractions:

(a)  2 5/8 = _____
(b)  1 3/8 = _____
(c)  2 6/7 = _____
(d)  4 5/9 = _____

**25**

numerator
denominator
same

**25**

The numerator and denominator of a fraction are called the *terms* of that fraction. Sometimes when we work with a fraction, we must change its terms. For example, we can change the terms of a fraction by multiplying or by dividing *both* terms by the same number—a process called *finding equivalent fractions.* In finding equivalent fractions, we must multiply or divide both the

_____ and the _____ by the _____ number.

**26**

value

**26**

Finding an equivalent fraction does not alter the value of the fractional parts. The numbers in the numerator and denominator are changed, but the _____ of the fractional parts remains the same.

**27**

multiply

**27**

One way of making a number larger is to multiply it by another number. If we wished to find an equivalent fraction in which both terms are larger, we could _____ both terms by the same number.

**28**

divide
the same number

**28**

Multiplication makes a number larger; division makes it smaller. If we need to find an equivalent fraction in which both terms are smaller, we could _____ both terms by _____ .

**29**

multiply
divide

**29**

When we want to find an equivalent fraction in which both terms are larger than those in the original fraction, we can _____ by any number. But when we want an equivalent fraction in which the terms are smaller, we must _____ by a number that will go *evenly* into both the numerator and the denominator of the original fraction.

**30**

**30**

Finding an equivalent fraction in which both terms are smaller is sometimes called "reducing the fraction to lower terms." When we reduce a fraction to

equivalent
smaller

lower terms, we are finding a(n)
_____ fraction that is _____
_____ .

**31**

multiply

## 31

Now you can see that finding an equivalent fraction can involve either reducing the fraction or enlarging it, depending on whether you divide or _____ both terms by the same number.

**32**

(a) 3/5
(b) 4/5
(c) cannot be further reduced
(d) 4/5
(e) cannot be further reduced

## 32

For practice in finding equivalent fractions in which both terms are smaller, reduce the following fractions to their lowest terms:

(a)  9/15 _____
(b)  12/15 _____
(c)  5/8 _____
(d)  16/20 _____
(e)  3/16 _____

**33**

gr. 6/6=1 grain

## 33

You're ready now to get down to the business of adding fractions. Try this problem to see how well you do: A patient has received the following doses of a certain drug—gr. 1/3, gr. 1/6 and gr. ss. (You'll recall that ss. means 1/2.) What is the total amount of drug the patient received?_____ .

The addition of fractions involves several steps. If you got the answer to Frame 33 right, you must already understand these steps and you should, therefore, go on to Frame 49. If you missed the question, or if you're unsure about it, continue with Frame 34 for a review of the addition of fractions.

**34**

numerators

**34**

When we add fractions we must remember that we are adding parts of a unit that has been divided. The numerators indicate the parts taken from the unit. In adding fractions, only the _____ are added.

**35**

value

**35**

Another point to remember is that the way in which a unit has been divided determines the value or size of the parts taken. If you divided a tablet into 4 parts, and then divided a similar tablet into 2 parts, you would not consider all parts of both tablets to be of equal _____.

**36**

**36**

The denominator of a fraction shows the way in which a unit has been divided. If you wished to add the parts of several units, you would have to make sure first that all of the units had been divided in the same way. Another way of saying

denominators

this is: The _____ of all the fractions to be added together must be the same.

**37**

denominator

**37**

There are two steps in the addition of fractions of like denominators. First, add the numerators, and secondly place the sum of all the numerators over the _____ , which is the same for all the fractions being added.

**38**

5/4 grains, or
  gr. 1 1/4

**38**

You use these two steps in the addition of fractions when you need to know the total amount of a drug the patient has received. For instance, Mrs. Jones received gr. 3/4 of a drug at 10:00 a.m., gr. 1/4 at 2:00 p.m., and gr. 1/4 at 5:00 p.m. How much of the drug did she receive during the day? (Write your answer both as an improper fraction and as a mixed number.) _____ .

**39**

equivalent
denominator

**39**

But what happens when the denominators are not all alike? Then you must change the fractions to _____ fractions, so that all the denominators are the same. The first step in doing this is called finding the "lowest common _____ ."

**40**

common

**40**

We know that a denominator that is "common to" all the denominators in the fractions being added must have some similarity to, or something in _____ with, all these denominators.

**41**

denominators

**41**

The one thing it must have in common with these denominators is *divisibility*. In other words, it must be a number that can be evenly divided by the _____ of all fractions being added.

**42**

15

**42**

When you are working with small fractions, finding the lowest common denominator can usually be done just by inspection. Look at this column of fractions:

3/5
4/5
2/3

The lowest common denominator (the L.C.D.) of the fractions in this column is

_____ .

**43**

**43**

If you chose 15 for the L.C.D. in Frame 42, you were right. This number can be divided evenly by the denominators 5 and 3 in the column of fractions. It is also the lowest possible number that is divisible by all the _____ in the column.

denominators

NOTE: When the L.C.D. cannot be determined by inspection, we must resort to mechanical means to determine the number. Because you will almost always works with small fractions, we have not included this problem in the program.

**44**

3
9

**44**

When you have determined the L.C.D., you must change all the fractions being added so that each one will have the L.C.D. figure as its denominator. We know that when the denominator is changed the numerator must also be changed, so that the value of the fraction will remain the same.

There is a quick and easy way to find the numerator. Let's say our fraction is 3/5 and the L.C.D. is 15:

First:     $15 \div 5 =$ _____
Second:    $3 \times 3 =$ _____

**45**

9/15

**45**

The number 9 is our new numerator. This is placed over the L.C.D., and 3/5 becomes _____ .
(fraction)

**46**

$15 \div 3 = 5$
$5 \times 2 = 10$
$10/15$

**46**

We'll try this one more time with the fraction 2/3. Our L.C.D. is 15.

*First:* the L.C.D. is divided by the denominator:

_____ ÷ _____ = _____

*Second:* multiply this number by the numerator of the fraction:

_____ × _____ = _____

We have now changed 2/3 to_____.

(fraction)

**47**

$9/15$
$12/15$
$10/15$

**47**

For our original column of fractions, the L.C.D. is 15. How would the fractions look after changing them so that all the denominators are 15?

$3/5 = $ _____
$4/5 = $ _____
$2/3 = $ _____

**48**

$31/15$

**48**

Now you can add these fractions just as you would add any other fractions with like denominators. Thus, 9/15 + 12/15 + 10/15=_____.

## 49

(a) 14/10 (or 7/5)
(b) 41/24
(c) 6/4 (or 3/2)
(d) 19/12

## 49

Test yourself on the following problems to be sure that you understand the addition of fractions:

(a)  1/2
     3/5
    +3/10

(b)  1/2
     3/8
    +5/6

(c)  1/2
     1/4
    +3/4

(d)  1/6
     2/3
    +3/4

## 50

5 3/8 quarts

## 50

If you understand the addition of fractions, you should have no trouble with the addition of mixed numbers, because when we add mixed numbers we are simply adding whole numbers and fractions. See how well you can do with the following situations: A head nurse is checking her supply of sterile saline solution. In one bottle she has 1 1/2 quarts, in another bottle 2 3/4 quarts, and in a third bottle 1 1/8 quarts.

She has a total of _____ quart(s) of saline solution.

If you worked the problem in Frame 50 without difficulty, go on to Frame 58. If you were not sure how to work the problem, go on to Frame 51 for a review of adding mixed numbers.

**51**

right

A column of mixed numbers is very similar to a column of whole numbers with two digits, for there are actually two columns to be added. When we add either mixed numbers or numbers of two or more digits, we always add the column on the · left/right · first.

**52**

**52**

right
fractions

In a mixed number, the fraction is written to the right of the whole number. Since we always begin by adding the column on the _____ , our first step in the addition of *mixed numbers* is to add the · whole numbers/fractions ·

**53**

**53**

fractions
whole numbers

When we add columns of mixed numbers, we add the _____ first and then the _____ _____ .

**54**

**54**

mixed
whole numbers

Our third step is to add the sum of the fractions to the sum of the whole numbers. If the sum of the fractions is an improper fraction—as it often is—we must change it to a _____ number before it is added to the sum of the _____ _____ .

**55**

15/8

---

**55**

Now let's use these steps in a problem involving the addition of mixed numbers. The column of mixed numbers is:

$$1\ 3/4$$
$$2\ 5/8$$
$$\underline{+1\ 1/2}$$

The first step in adding these figures is to find the sum of the column of fractions, the column on the right. Before doing this, however, we must find the L.C.D. and change all the fractions to equivalent fractions, This gives us:

$$6/8$$
$$5/8$$
$$\underline{+4/8}$$

Thus _____ is your answer for the sum
    (fraction)
of the column of fractions.

---

**56**

1 7/8

---

**56**

We take the sum of the fractions and then change the resulting improper fraction to a mixed number.

$$15/8 = \underline{\hspace{2cm}}$$

---

**57**

---

**57**

Now we must find the sum of the whole numbers $(1 + 2 + 1 = 4)$, and add this to the sum of the fractions (1 7/8):

$$\begin{array}{r} 4 \\ +1\ 7/8 \\ \hline \end{array}$$

5 7/8                Your answer: _____

58

**58**

(a)  6  6/15
(b) 10  7/8
(c) 15 11/24
(d)  8  5/8

Add the following mixed numbers. Be sure to find the L.C.D. and to change all the fractions to equivalent fractions of like denominators before you add them.

$$\begin{array}{ll} \text{(a)} & 1\ 2/5 \\ & 3\ 2/3 \\ & +1\ 5/15 \\ \hline \end{array} \qquad \begin{array}{ll} \text{(b)} & 4\ 1/4 \\ & 1\ 1/2 \\ & +5\ 1/8 \\ \hline \end{array}$$

$$\begin{array}{ll} \text{(c)} & 8\ 1/3 \\ & 4\ 3/8 \\ & +2\ 3/4 \\ \hline \end{array} \qquad \begin{array}{ll} \text{(d)} & 1\ 4/16 \\ & 2\ 3/4 \\ & +4\ 5/8 \\ \hline \end{array}$$

59

**59**

gr. 1/8

Now let us see how well you remember the subtraction of fractions. One of your patients is to receive gr. 1/8 of morphine sulfate, and the only dosage on hand is an ampule containing gr. 1/4. Since morphine is a narcotic, you are required to account for the amount you do not use for the patient.

gr. 1/4 — gr. 1/8 = _____ grain(s)

If you answered the question in Frame 59 correctly, go on to Frame 64. If you did not understand how to do it, go on to Frame 60 for a review of the subtraction of fractions.

## 60

common
subtract

### 60

When we add fractions, we can only add the numerators of fractions with like denominators. The same rule applies when we subtract fractions.

In the subtraction of fractions we must have a _____ denominator before we can _____ one numerator from the other.

## 61

2/8 (or 1/4)

### 61

Suppose that you wanted to subtract 2/8 from 4/8. That's easy, because your denominators are the same and the numbers in the numerator are so small that you can work the problem in your head. Your answer is_____.

## 62

5/16

### 62

Now let's subtract 2/8 from 9/16. The answer is · 7/8 / 5/16 ·

## 63

### 63

Remember that we subtract only the numerators, and that all the fractions must have a common denominator. We

equivalent
numerators

must first find the L.C.D. and then change to _____ fractions before we can subtract the _____.

**64**

(a) 3/16
(b) 1/2
(c) 1/4
(d) 2/5

**64**

Just for practice, subtract the following fractions:

(a)  11/16
   − 8/16
   ―――――

(b)  3/5
   −1/10
   ―――――

(c)  2/5
   −3/20
   ―――――

(d)  9/10
   −2/4
   ―――――

**65**

gr. 1 3/4

**65**

The subtraction of mixed numbers may well be easy for you. Let's suppose that you have given a patient gr. 1 3/4 from an ampule that contained gr. iiiss. of a certain drug, and that you must account for the amount left in the ampule. When you subtract the amount given from the amount on hand, you will have a remainder of_____grain(s).

If your answer to the question in Frame 65 was wrong, and you would like to review the subtraction of mixed numbers, go on to Frame 66. If you are sure that you can do such problems easily, go on to Frame 69.

fractions

Remember that when we add mixed numbers we add the fractions first. The same rule applies to the subtraction of mixed numbers. Our first step, then, is to subtract the _____ in the mixed number.

whole number

Once again we can see the similarity between mixed numbers and numbers having two digits. When the fraction in the subtrahend (bottom number) is larger than the fraction in the minuend (top number), we "borrow" from the column on the left. In subtracting mixed numbers we sometimes must borrow from the · whole number / fraction column ·

1 2/3

Let's say our problem is:
$$4 \ 1/3$$
$$-2 \ 2/3$$

We have changed it to:
$$3 \ 4/3$$
$$-2 \ 2/3$$

The answer is: _____

## 69

(a) 2 9/16
(b) 9 5/8
(c) 1 1/2
(d) 3 3/10

## 69

Work these subtraction problems for practice:

$$
\begin{array}{cc}
\text{(a)} & 4\ 5/8 \\
& -2\ 1/16 \\
\hline
\end{array}
\qquad
\begin{array}{cc}
\text{(b)} & 25\ 1/8 \\
& -15\ 1/2 \\
\hline
\end{array}
$$

$$
\begin{array}{cc}
\text{(c)} & 6\ 1/3 \\
& -4\ 5/6 \\
\hline
\end{array}
\qquad
\begin{array}{cc}
\text{(d)} & 5\ 9/10 \\
& -2\ 3/5 \\
\hline
\end{array}
$$

## 70

1/2 × 1/4

## 70

It is often necessary to multiply fractions as you prepare medications for administration; and you can easily make a serious mistake in dosage if you do not understand exactly what you are doing when you multiply fractions.

First of all, it is necessary to recognize that 1/2 of 1/4 is a problem in *multiplication.* To find the answer, we would write the problem:

———— × ————

## 71

multiply
1/300

## 71

We have said that the word "of" in a problem involving fractions tells us that we must _____. In a situation in which the nurse must give 1/2 of 1/150, should she administer 1/75 or 1/300?_____.

If you got the right answer to the question in Frame 71, go on to Frame 75. If not, continue with Frame 72 for a fuller explanation.

**72**

2 × 3

**72**

Multiplying fractions involves first multiplying the numerators together and then multiplying the denominators together. To multiply 2/3 × 3/4, we would first multiply_____ × _____ to find the product of the numerators.

**73**

denominators

**73**

Our next step is to multiply 3 × 4, to find the product of the _____
_____.

**74**

6/12
1/2

**74**

After we have found the product of the numerators and the product of the denominators, we reduce the fraction to its lowest terms:

2/3 × 3/4 = _____
(fraction)

This fraction can be reduced to_____.

**75**

**75**

To simplify the multiplication of fractions, we can divide any numerator and denominator by the same number. This

divide
the same

is called "cancellation." When we "cancel," we _____ any numerator and any denominator by_____ _____ number.

**76**

2

**76**

Let's simplify the problem 2/3 × 3/4 by cancelling:

$$\frac{2}{3} \times \frac{3}{4}$$

You can see that both 2 and 4 can be evenly divided by_____.

**77**

3

**77**

Now your problem is changed to look like this:

$$\frac{\overset{1}{\cancel{2}}}{3} \times \frac{3}{\underset{2}{\cancel{4}}}$$

You can also see that the numerator 3 and denominator 3 can both be evenly divided by_____.

**78**

1/2

**78**

Thus, dividing the 3 in the numerator and the 3 in the denominator each by 3, our problem looks like this:

$$\frac{\overset{1}{\cancel{2}}}{\underset{1}{\cancel{3}}} \times \frac{\overset{1}{\cancel{3}}}{\underset{2}{\cancel{4}}} = \frac{1}{1} \times \frac{1}{2}$$

Multiplying this out gives us _____
(fraction)

**79**

1/6

**79**

If a patient is to receive 1/2 of an ampule of Pantopon that contains gr. 1/3, you should know that the patient is to receive _____ grain(s).

**80**

$$\frac{3}{5} \times \frac{14}{1}$$

**80**

Multiplying fractions by whole numbers really isn't any different from multiplying fractions. All we need to do is write the whole number as the numerator and use 1 as the denominator. To multiply 3/5 × 14, we would write our problem like this (supply the missing denominator):

$$\frac{3}{5} \times \frac{14}{}$$

**81**

600

**81**

If 2/5 of a 1500-calorie diet consists of protein, we can calculate that protein provides _____ calories in the diet.

**82**

8/5
15/4

**82**

The multiplication of mixed numbers is just as easy if you change the mixed numbers to improper fractions, and then multiply the fractions.

To multiply 1 3/5 × 3 3/4, you must first change 1 3/5 to _____ and 3 3/4 to _____.

**83**

5 5/8

**83**

Now let's see how you would use the multiplication of mixed numbers in a situation. Your instructor adds 1 1/2 ampules of a drug to some intravenous fluid. Each ampule contains 3 3/4 grains of the drug.

Administering 1 1/2 ampules containing 3 3/4 grains each would give the patient a total of _____ grain(s) of the drug.

**84**

5 1/4 quarts

**84**

You must instruct a patient's family to prepare a 3 1/2 days' supply of supplemental feeding. The daily amount necessary for this patient is 1 1/2 quarts.

The total amount of supplemental feeding would be _____ quart(s).

**85**

(a) 1/6
(b) 30/7
(c) 1/75
(d) 75/8

**85**

For review in multiplying several different types of fractions, work the following problems:

(a) 4/12 × 3/6 _____
(b) 15 × 2/7 _____
(c) 1/150 × 2 _____
(d) 2 1/2 × 3 6/8 _____

**86**

**86**

Dividing fractions can be a little tricky, but if you remember the first step the rest is easy. When we divide fractions we

3/4

must first *invert the divisor.* The divisor is the number you "divide by." If you have 7/8 divided by 3/4, should you invert 7/8 or 3/4?

**87**

4/3

**87**

To "invert" means to turn upside down or to reverse positions. When you invert 3/4 it becomes _____.

**88**

multiplication

**88**

When you invert the divisor, you reverse the process of division and change it into its exact opposite, which is multiplication. Inverting the fraction you want to divide by changes the problem from one of division to one of _____.

**89**

1/2

**89**

Let's say that you must divide 1/6 by 1/3 to determine how much of a fractional dose to give. You must write your problem as 1/6 ÷ 1/3. After inverting the divisor and multiplying the fractions, the answer is_____.

**90**

improper
fractions

**90**

Dividing mixed numbers presents no problem, because the mixed numbers can be changed to _____ fractions. After you have made this change, the problem is simply a matter of dividing the_____.

## 91

(a) 4/45
(b) 7/2
(c) 152/33
(d) 1/2

## 91

Just for practice, work the following problems in division:

(a) $1/15 \div 3/4$ = _____

(b) $2/3 \div 4/21$ = _____

(c) $6\ 1/3 \div 1\ 3/8$ = _____

(d) $1/300 \div 1/150$ = _____

# Post-test on the Apothecaries' System

A. Complete the following table of equivalents:

1. _____ drams = 1 ounce
2. _____ ounces = 1 pint
3. _____ pints = 1 quart
4. _____ ounces = 1 quart
5. _____ quarts = 1 gallon

B. Write the correct abbreviations for the following:

6. gallon _____
7. quart _____
8. pint _____
9. ounce _____
10. dram _____
11. grain _____

C. Write the correct symbols for the following:

12. ounce _____
13. dram _____
14. minim _____

D. Write the following dosages as they would be read aloud, that is, "two and one-half drams."

15. ℨ iiss. _____
16. ℨ iv _____
17. ℨ ii _____
18. ℥ ss. _____
19. ℥ viii _____
20. ♏ xiii _____
21. ♏ vii _____
22. gr. viiss _____
23. gr. xx _____
24. gr. xv _____

E. Chart the following dosages using the correct symbols, abbreviations, and numbers:

25. Three ounces of mineral oil: _____
26. One and one-half drams of cascara: _____
27. Fifteen minims of tincture of belladonna:_____
28. One-half dram of Elixir of Donnatal: _____
29. Five grains of aspirin: _____

F. Situations:

30. A solution of 3% aluminum acetate is to be prepared for use as cold compresses. If 2 patients on the unit are receiving the compresses 4 times daily and 8 ounces of solution is needed for each application, _____ quart(s) of solution must be prepared for a one-day supply. This is the same as _____ gallon(s).

31. Milk of magnesia is a laxative that is used frequently. The nurse on postpartum has 18 patients who are to receive 1 ounce of the medication this p.m. If the stock bottle contains one pint, will there be sufficient medication for all the patients?_____.

32. Mrs. Hamer received Sodium Butisol gr. 1/4 at 10:00 a.m., gr. 3/4 at 2:00 p.m. and gr. ss. at 6:00 p.m. The recommended daily dosage as a sedative should not exceed 2 grains daily. Did she receive more than the usual daily dosage?_____.

33. What would be the total number of grains received by a patient who is given gr. ss, gr. 1/6, and gr. 3 3/4 of a certain drug?_____.

34. The doctor has ordered Dilaudid gr. 1/64 and the ampule contains gr. 1/32. _____grain(s) of medication will remain in the ampule after the dosage has been withdrawn.

35. Let's suppose that a patient is given gr. 3 3/4 from an ampule containing gr. viiss. The amount left in the ampule will be gr. _____.

36. If you were to give a patient 1/2 of a tablet that contains gr. 1/4, how many grains would the patient receive?_____.

37. If you gave a patient 2 tablets containing gr. 1/150 each, would the patient receive a total of gr. 1/300 or gr. 1/75?_____

38. The patient is to receive Atropine gr. 1/100. If it is available in tablets containing gr. 1/200, you would give the patient _____tablet(s).

39. Mr. Martin has received Papaverine gr. iss. five times today. A total of _____grains has been given.

# PART THREE

# THE
# HOUSEHOLD
# SYSTEM

**1**

teaspoon
tablespoon

**1**

We have said that when drugs are administered in the home it is often necessary to measure them in some household article such as a teaspoon or tablespoon. These articles are not always standard in size, however, and they should be used only if absolutely necessary.

Two units of measure in the household system are the_____ and _____ .

**2**

4 teaspoonfuls

**2**

When medications are ordered according to the household system, it would be best to use a medicine glass graduated in household units. Look at the drawing below.

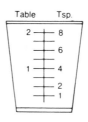

_____ teaspoonfuls = 1 tablespoonful

**3**

**3**

This glass (pictured front and back) is a 1 ounce glass.

1 ounce glass.

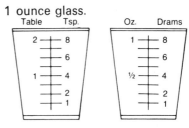

2 tablespoonfuls

You can see that there are approximately _____ tablespoonfuls in 1 ounce.

**4**

**4**

1 dram

Look at the drawing in Frame 3. A teaspoonful is approximately equivalent to what unit of measure in the apothecaries' system? _____.

# Post-test on the Household System

## A. Situations:

1. A clinic patient has been instructed to take 1 table-spoonful of Kaon elixir twice daily. He is receiving the average daily dosage of _____ ounce(s) per day.

2. The doctor has ordered 1 teaspoonful of Elixir of Donnatal to be given before each meal and at bedtime. The patient is given a total of _____ tablespoonful(s) daily.

3. The order reads Mineral Oil ℥ ss. This could be measured as _____ tablespoonful(s).

4. A patient is to receive two teaspoonfuls of Maalox four times each day. The drug is supplied in 12 ounce bottles. How many bottles will she need to take home for a two weeks' supply? _____ .

# PART FOUR

# THE
# METRIC
# SYSTEM

# UNIT I

# Review of Decimals

**1**

measurement

**1**

The metric system is the system of
_____ that you will
find most useful, because it is the one
most frequently used in the official
listings of drugs. The metric system is
very logically organized, and it uses
decimal numbers for expressing various
amounts. This makes it necessary to have
a full understanding of decimals before
we begin to study the metric system.

**2**

10
10

**2**

The word decimal comes from the Latin
word for "ten." The decimal system is
based on the number 10. A decimal
fraction is a fraction whose denominator
is the number _____ or some power of
the number _____.

**3**

denominator
decimal

**3**

We have said that, besides the number 10
itself, the _____ of a _____
fraction can also be a power of 10.

The word "power" in this sense means a
number multiplied by itself a certain

number of times. For example, 10 × 10 × 10 = 1000; and therefore 1000 is known as the third power of 10.

**4**

power

**4**

We can use the decimal system to express mixed numbers or fractions, but the denominator of a decimal fraction must be the number 10 or some _____ of 10, such as 100, 1000, or 10,000.

**5**

75/100 (Because the denominator is a power of 10.)

**5**

Which of the following fractions could also be written as a decimal fraction?

2/3         75/100         10/25

**6**

left
right

**6**

There are three parts to a decimal: the integer (whole number), the decimal point, and the decimal fraction. Look at their relative positions in the drawing:

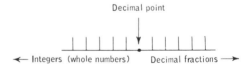

If you wanted to write the mixed number 1 5/10 as a decimal fraction, you would write the whole number 1 to the · left/right · of the decimal point, and the fraction 5/10 to the · left/right · of the decimal point.

**7**

decrease

**7**

The position of a number in relation to the decimal point is called the place value of the number. In the drawing, you can see that decimal fractions · decrease/increase · in value as the number moves farther to the right of the decimal point.

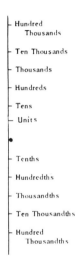

**8**

increases

**8**

Just as the decimal fraction has a definite value by virtue of its position, the integer also has a place value—but in exactly the opposite direction. As the whole number moves farther to the left of the decimal point, the value of the integer · increases/decreases.

**9**

thousandths

**9**

The place value or position of a number in relation to the decimal point gives the decimal number its place name.

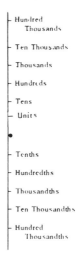

- Hundred Thousands
- Ten Thousands
- Thousands
- Hundreds
- Tens
- Units
- •
- Tenths
- Hundredths
- Thousandths
- Ten Thousandths
- Hundred Thousandths

A number in the third position to the right of the decimal point would have the place name _____.

**10**

thousandths

**10**

The number 0.365 would therefore be read as "three hundred and sixty-five _____."

**11**

tenths

**11**

A number in the first position to the right of the decimal point would have the place name _____.

**12**

two tenths

**12**

A decimal written as 0.2 is read as

_____  _____ .

**13**

eight hundredths

**13**

A number in the second position to the right of the decimal point would have the place name "hundredths." Thus, 0.08 is read as _____

_____ .

**14**

0.365

**14**

To eliminate confusion from overlooking the decimal point and reading a decimal fraction as a whole number, a zero is placed to the left of the decimal point when there is no integer in the decimal. Three hundred sixty-five thousandths should be written as _____ .

**15**

0.75

**15**

A decimal that reads seventy-five hundredths should be written as _____ .

**16**

fourteen and
   three hundred
   sixty-five
   thousandths

**16**

The number to the left of the decimal point is read just as you would read any whole number. The decimal point itself is read as "and". Thus you would read the figure 14.365 as "_____

_____ ."

**17**

one and twenty-
five hundredths

**17**

A physician's order written as 1.25 mg. of a certain drug should be read as _____ milligrams.

**18**

are

**18**

We have said that the decimal fraction takes its value from its position in relation to the decimal point. If this is true, then 0.5 and 0.50 · are/are not · of equal value.

**19**

value

**19**

You will recall that reducing a common fraction does not change its value. For instance, 50/100 can be reduced to 5/10 without altering the value of the fraction. Therefore, changing 0.5 to 0.50 does not alter the _____ of the decimal fraction.

**20**

does not
change

**20**

If 0.5 and 0.50 are of equal value, then it should be possible to annex zeros to the decimal fraction without changing its value. By "annexing zeros" we mean placing additional zeros to the right of the fraction number. Placing extra zeros to the right of a decimal fraction · changes/does not change · the value of the fraction.

**21**

$$\begin{array}{r} 0.30 \\ +0.25 \\ \hline 0.55 \end{array}$$

**21**

This trick of annexing zeros comes in very handy when adding decimals. The numbers to be added are placed so that the decimal points are lined up directly under one another, and then zeros can be annexed when they are needed.

Show how you would write out the problem 0.3 + 0.25:

$$+ \underline{\hspace{2cm}}$$

Your answer: _____

**22**

$$\begin{array}{r} 3.500 \\ 0.250 \\ +0.001 \\ \hline 3.751 \end{array}$$

**22**

How would you annex zeros to add 3.5, 0.25, and 0.001?

$$+ \underline{\hspace{2cm}}$$

Your answer: _____

**23**

decimal points

**23**

In the subtraction of decimals, we line up the decimal points just as we do for addition. Whenever we subtract decimals, we should annex zeros so that the _____ _____ are directly under one another.

**24**

**24**

When we subtract decimals, we write the problem just as we would for whole numbers. The decimal point in the remainder (that is, the answer) is lined up with the decimal points in the minuend and the subtrahend.

Show how you would write out the problem 2.5 − 0.08:

2.50
−0.08
‾‾‾‾
2.42

Your answer: _____

## 25

12.25
− 7.50
‾‾‾‾
4.75

## 25

Let's suppose that the nurse in charge must order medication for a patient who is leaving the hospital in the morning. She has in the medicine cabinet 12.25 mg. of the drug, and the patient will receive 7.5 mg. during the night. In order to determine how much of the drug will be left for the patient to take home in the morning, the nurse must subtract 7.5 mg from 12.25 mg. Her answer is _____ mg.

## 26

decimal point

## 26

The multiplication of decimals is easy if we remember that the only thing that distinguishes decimal numbers from whole numbers is the decimal point. The multiplication of decimal numbers is done in exactly the same way as the multiplication of whole numbers, except for the placing of the _____ _____ in the product.

**27**

three

**27**

After multiplying our decimal numbers, we must determine the proper location of the decimal point in the product. This is done simply by counting the total number of decimal places in the multiplier and the multiplicand. Thus, if there are two decimal places in the multiplier and one decimal place in the multiplicand, there will be a total of _____ decimal places in the product.

**28**

right

**28**

When we say decimal places we mean the number of places to the right of the decimal point. If you have a total of three decimal places to account for in the product, then you must have three numbers to the · left/right · of the decimal point.

**29**

seven

**29**

Let's suppose that we need to multiply 0.0004 times 0.356. After we have multiplied the numbers, we must place the decimal point so as to have a total of _____ decimal places to the right of the decimal point in the product.

**30**

**30**

To multiply 0.60 × 2.49, we would proceed just as we would for multiplying whole numbers, and then determine the location of the decimal point by counting the total number of decimal places in the multiplier and multiplicand. If our product for $0.60 \times 2.49$ is 14940, then the decimal point is placed between the _____ and the _____.

between 1
and 4

## 31

.31

zeros

Sometimes, when we multiply decimals, the product contains fewer figures than we have decimal places. In this case we must prefix as many zeros as necessary. If, for example, the product is 365 and we need five decimal places, we would have to place two _____ in front of the 365.

## 32

## 32

in front of

Now our 365 becomes 0.00365 because we have prefixed two zeros in order to have enough decimal places. Prefixing zeros means placing the required number of zeros · in front of/behind · the product.

## 33

## 33

three

When we multiply decimals, we know that we must finish with a definite number of decimal places in the product. In the problem $0.2 \times 0.03$, the product is six thousandths. Therefore we must account for _____ decimal places in the product.

**34**

two
0.006

**34**

Since we know that we must account for three decimal places, we prefix _____ zeros to the decimal fraction. The six thousandths is therefore written as the decimal number _____.

**35**

0.000028

**35**

After multiplying 0.014 × 0.002, we will need six decimal places in the product. The problem would be written:

$$\begin{array}{r} 0.014 \\ \times\,0.002 \\ \hline \end{array}$$

Your answer: _____

**36**

one

**36**

The multiplication of a decimal by the number 10 or any multiple of 10 is easy. Each time we move the decimal point one place to the right, we have multiplied by 10. If we wished to multiply 27.3 by 10, we would move the decimal point _____ place(s) to the right.

**37**

**37**

If we multiply by 10 each time that we move the decimal point one place to the right, then moving the decimal point three places to the right would be the same as 10 × 10 × 10, or 1000 times the number. To multiply $6.3 \times 1000$, all you need to do is move the decimal point _____ places to the right.

three

## 38

two
425

### 38

Moving the decimal point to the right is a short-cut for multiplying by 10 or any power of 10. A quick way to multiply 4.25 by 100 is to move the decimal point _____ place(s) to the right. The product of $4.25 \times 100$ is _____ .

## 39

divisor: 6
dividend: 30
quotient: 5

### 39

Decimal numbers are divided the same way whole numbers are divided. The only difference is that you must be sure to account for the decimal point. An ordinary problem in division is made up of three parts, which are named as follows:

$$\text{divisor } \overline{)\, \text{dividend}}^{\text{quotient}}$$

In the problem $30 \div 6$, the divisor is _____ , and the dividend is _____ ; the quotient (that is, the answer) would be

_____ .

## 40

0.5

### 40

In dividing with decimals, it is only necessary to remember to keep the decimal point in the quotient directly above the decimal point in the dividend. Therefore, in the problem $3.5 \div 7$, the quotient would be _____ .

## 41

whole number

**41**

One important point to remember in the division of decimals is that the divisor must always be a whole number. In a problem in which the divisor is a decimal number, you must move the decimal point to the right as many places as necessary to change the decimal number into a_____ _____.

## 42

two

right

**42**

Whole numbers are always written to the left of the decimal point. To change 0.46 to a whole number, you would move the decimal point _____places to the _____.

## 43

divisor
  (0.46 becomes
  46)
dividend
  (3.22 becomes
  322)

**43**

Since moving the decimal point changes the place value of a number, we cannot move the decimal point in the divisor without also moving it the same number of places in the dividend. Before we can divide 3.22 by 0.46, we must move the decimal point two places to the right in both the_____and the_____.

## 44

**44**

If we move the decimal point in the divisor we must also move it in the dividend. The decimal point in the quotient is placed above the decimal point in the dividend after it has been moved.

In the problem $3.22 \div 0.46$, the decimal point is placed to the · left/right of the 7 in the quotient.

right

**45**

zeros
2500.0

**45**

In some problems of division, the dividend is a whole number but the divisor is a decimal number. When the dividend is a whole number, it is understood that the decimal point is located to the right of that number (thus 25 could be read as 25.0).

In a problem in which the divisor is 0.05 and the dividend is 25, we must move the decimal point two places to the right in both the divisor and the dividend. Since there are no numbers to the right of the whole number 25, we must annex two _____ before we can move the decimal point to the right.

After moving the decimal point in the divisor, 0.05 becomes 05.0 (which is the same as 5); and after moving the decimal point in the dividend, the whole number 25 becomes _____ .

500

After we have annexed the necessary zeros and moved the decimal points, our problem looks like this:

$$05. \overline{) 2500.0}$$

The quotient is _____ .

4

To divide 10 by 2.5 we must change our divisor to a whole number, annex zeros to the dividend, and move the decimal point. The problem is written:

$$25. \overline{) 100}$$

The quotient is _____ .

80

Now let's say that we need to divide 280 by 3.5. Move the decimal points and find the quotient. Your answer is _____ .

0.06

Sometimes when we divide decimals we find that our divisor is larger than our dividend. When this happens, we can annex as many zeros as we need in the dividend, without moving the decimal point in either the divisor or the dividend.

In the problem 0.3 ÷ 5, we change the 0.3 to 0.30 and divide as we would for whole numbers. Thus, 0.30 ÷ 5 = _____ .

**50**

0.0005

**50**

Suppose that we had to divide 0.006 by 12. We know that we must annex zeros and divide just as we would for whole numbers, being sure to place the decimal point in the quotient directly above the decimal point in the dividend.

The quotient of $0.006 \div 12$ is _____.

**51**

left

**51**

Dividing is the opposite of multiplying. A short cut for multiplying a number by 10 or powers of 10 is to move the decimal point to the right. A quick and easy way to divide by 10 or powers of 10 is to move the decimal point to the

_____ .

**52**

two

**52**

To divide 10.5 by 100, we can take a short cut and simply move the decimal point _____ places to the left.

**53**

0.02287

**53**

The problem $22.87 \div 1000$ can be easily solved by moving the decimal point to the left. Our answer is _____ .

**54**

**54**

A common fraction can easily be changed to a decimal fraction. For instance, 4/5 is the same as $4 \div 5$. Dividing

4 by 5 is no problem because we can annex as many zeros as necessary to the dividend.

To change 4/5 to a decimal, we write the problem as:

$$5 \overline{)\ 4.0}$$

0.8    The answer is _____ .

**55**

0.6    If we needed to change 3/5 to a decimal fraction, we would write our problem as $3 \div 5$.

The answer is _____ .

**56**

right    Mixed numbers also can be changed to decimals without difficulty. The integer (whole number) is simply written to the left of the decimal point. The common fraction, however, must be changed to a decimal fraction. Decimal fractions are always written to the _____ of the decimal point.

**57**

12.5    The mixed number 12 1/2 contains an integer and a common fraction. This mixed number can be written as the decimal number _____ .

## 58

3.75

## 58

If we changed the common fraction in the mixed number 3 3/4 to a decimal fraction, and wrote the mixed number as a decimal, we would have _____.

## 59

5/100

## 59

To reverse the process and write a decimal fraction as a common fraction, we simply write the fraction as we would read it aloud. For instance, 0.05 is read as "five hundredths." Written as a common fraction, 0.05 would be _____.

fraction

## 60

33/1000

## 60

We read 0.033 as thirty-three thousandths. We write it as the common fraction _____.

## 61

(a) 1 1/4
(b) 75/10000
(c) 64/100
(d) 0.02
(e) 0.375
(f) 0.05

## 61

You will encounter many situations in which you must write decimal fractions as common fractions, and in which you must change common fractions to decimal fractions. For practice, work the following problems:

(a) 1.25   = _____ (mixed number)
(b) 0.0075 = _____ (common fraction)
(c) 0.64   = _____ (common fraction)
(d) 1/50   = _____ (decimal fraction)
(e) 3/8    = _____ (decimal fraction)
(f) 1/20   = _____ (decimal fraction)

# UNIT II

# Units of Measure in the Metric System

**1**

secondary

**1**

Now you should be ready to learn the units of measure in the metric system. These consist of the primary units (the ones on which the system is based) and the secondary units (which are derived from the primary units). We are chiefly concerned with only two primary units in the metric system: the liter and the gram.

In the metric system, all units of measure derived from the liter and the gram are_____ units.

**2**

grams

**2**

The liter is the primary unit used in measuring liquid capacity; the gram is the primary unit used in measuring solid weight. A solid drug would therefore be weighed in · liters/grams ·

**3**

**3**

Because some liquids are much more viscous and therefore heavier than other liquids that might occupy the same amount of space, we usually speak of weighing solids and measuring liquids.

measured in
liters

You would expect a saline solution to be
· weighed in grams/measured in liters ·

**4**

liter

**4**

We have said that secondary units are
derived from primary units. The nomenclature used in medical science contains
many terms that are combinations of
prefixes or suffixes taken from Latin or
Greek. The naming of secondary units is
an example of this type of self-
explanatory nomenclature.

For example the prefix *milli-* means one-
thousandth. The secondary unit called
*milliliter* simply means one thousandth
of a _____.

**5**

1000 milliliters

**5**

If the word milliliter means one-
thousandth of a liter, then we know that
there are _____ milliliters in 1 liter.

**6**

milligram

**6**

The *milliliter* is a secondary unit of
measure because it is derived from the
primary unit, the liter. By adding the
prefix *milli-* to the primary unit *gram,*
we have another secondary unit; it is
called the _____.

**7**

gram

**7**

There are 1000 milligrams in 1 gram. Another way of expressing this is to say: 1 milligram equals 0.001 _____.

**8**

liter
gram
milliliter
milligram

**8**

The prefix *milli-* is used in naming secondary units of measure. Other prefixes may be used, but they are rarely applied in the calculation of dosage. Thus there are only really four units of measure which you will use regularly. These are the primary units: the _____ and the _____ and the secondary units: the _____ and the _____.

**9**

microgram

**9**

Another unit of measure that is sometimes used in pharmacology but does not involve conversion by the nurse is the microgram. This unit is one-thousandth of a milligram. The smallest unit of solid measure in the metric system is one-thousandth of a milligram and is called a

_____.

**10**

milligram

**10**

A microgram is equivalent to one-thousandth of a _____.

# UNIT III

# Abbreviations and Numbers
# in the Metric System

**1**

liter

**1**

Now we should turn our attention to the abbreviations used for units of measure in the metric system. The abbreviation for liter is simply the first letter of the word; thus L. is the abbreviation for

_____.

**2**

ml.

**2**

The abbreviation for milliliter is the first letter of the prefix *milli-* plus the first letter of the word liter. The abbreviation for milliliter is _____.

**3**

the same as

**3**

Another abbreviation commonly used to designate one-thousandth of a liter is "cc." The cc. abbreviation stands for *cubic centimeter,* which is the amount of space occupied by one milliliter.

Thus 1 cc. is · smaller than/the same as/larger than · 1 milliliter.

**4**

metric
secondary
metric

**4**

The liter and the meter are both primary units of the _____ system; therefore, the milliliter and the centimeter are both _____ units of the _____ system.

**5**

grams

**5**

The abbreviation for gram is Gm. We use a capital G to avoid confusing Gm. with gr., the abbreviation for grain. A dosage of 0.1 Gm. means that the drug has been weighed and dispensed in · grains/grams ·

**6**

mg.

**6**

The abbreviation for milliliter is a combination of the first letter of the prefix *milli-* and the first letter of the word *liter.* The abbreviation for milligram is formed from a similar combination. The abbreviation for milligram is _____ .

**7**

mcg.

**7**

The abbreviation for microgram is a combination of mc. for the prefix micro and g. for the gram. The abbreviation for microgram is_____ .

**8**

0.25 mg.

**8**

We have said that the metric system is based on the decimal system. Thus, only decimals are used to designate amounts in the metric system. The decimal number is always written before an abbreviation for a unit of measure. Twenty-five hundredths of a milligram should be written as _____ .

**9**

0.1 mg.

**9**

If a physician orders one-tenth milligram of digitoxin, how would you chart the dosage, using the proper abbreviation and decimal numbers? _____ .

Did you remember to place a zero in front of the decimal point, to prevent errors in reading?

**10**

1.5 ml.

**10**

Sometimes we administer one and one-half milliliters by injection. This amount should be written as _____ .

**11**

gram

**11**

The dosage on a medicine card is written aspirin 0.3 Gm. You would read this as three-tenths of a _____ .

**12**

micrograms

**13**

1/2 cc.

**12**

The physician orders 10 mcg. of Vitamin B$_{12}$. The dosage is read as ten _____.

**13**

We have said that milliliters and cubic centimeters both express one-thousandth of a liter. Suppose that you were going to give a patient 0.5 ml. of a drug, and that your syringe was graduated in cc's. You would pull the plunger up to the line marked · 1/2 cc. / 2 cc. / 5 cc. ·

## UNIT IV

# Exchanging Weights Within the Metric System

**1**

1000 milligrams

**1**

Sometimes drugs are weighed and dispensed from the hospital pharmacy in grams, when the dosage is ordered in milligrams. In this instance you must be able to change the milligrams into grams.

Let's say that we have 2000 milligrams. We know that if 1000 milligrams are equal to 1 gram, then 2000 milligrams will be equal to 2 grams.

In changing the milligrams to grams, we divide the number of milligrams by 1000 because there are _____ milligrams in each gram.

**2**

three
left

**2**

There is an easy way to divide by 1000 when changing milligrams to grams. You will recall that if you wish to divide by 1000 you can simply move the decimal point three places to the left.

Now you can complete the following rule for changing milligrams to grams: To change milligrams to grams, move the decimal point _____ places to the _____ .

**3**

(a) 2 Gm.
(b) 0.5 Gm.
(c) 0.25 Gm.
(d) 0.1 Gm.

**3**

Change the following milligrams to grams:

(a) 2000 mg. = _____ Gm.
(b) 500 mg. = _____ Gm.
(c) 250 mg. = _____ Gm.
(d) 100 mg. = _____ Gm.

**4**

0.5 Gm.

**4**

Now you are ready to solve some problems of the kind that you may encounter as you prepare to give medications.

Suppose that the physician orders 500 mg. of a certain drug and that the drug is dispensed in 0.5 Gm. tablets. By moving the decimal point, you could determine that 500 mg. are equal to_____Gm.

**5**

1 tablet

**5**

Since 500 mg. are equal to 0.5 Gm., this patient should receive _____ tablet(s).

**6**

3 tablets

**6**

Let's say that a dose of 750 mg. of a certain drug has been ordered, and that the drug is dispensed in scored tablets of 0.25 Gm. each. The patient should be given _____ tablet(s).

1/4 tablet

Let's say that a physician orders 250 mg. of a medication that is dispensed in scored tablets of 1 Gm. each. The patient should receive _____ tablet(s).

scored

In Frame 7 the patient was given 1/4 of a tablet. This was done using a scored tablet; that is, one with grooves in it allowing for accurate fractional doses. Tablets that are grooved so that they can be broken into accurate halves or fourths are called _____ tablets.

100 mg.
2 tablets

Swallowing large numbers of tablets or capsules is difficult for some persons. To avoid unnecessary discomfort for your patient you should choose, from available drugs of varying strengths, the tablet or capsule that contains the amount most nearly equivalent to the dosage ordered for the patient.

If, for example, a patient is to receive 0.2 Gm. of a drug and there are available tablets of 10, 50, and 100 mg. each, which strength tablet would be most appropriate?_____. How many would you give?_____.

**10**

2 capsules

**10**

If a physician orders 4 mg. of a drug, and the label on the container reads 0.002 Gm. per capsule, you should give the patient _____ capsule(s).

**11**

0.1 Gm.
1 capsule

**11**

When you prepare to give 100 mg. of Seconal, you find that the drug is dispensed in 0.1 Gm. capsules. Since 100 mg. equals _____ Gm., you would give _____ capsule(s).

**12**

cannot

**12**

We have said that scored tablets can be divided to give accurate fractional doses. Capsules, on the other hand, are never scored for divided doses. You · can/cannot · administer less than one capsule.

**13**

three
right

**13**

It is only logical to recognize that if we can change milligrams to grams by moving the decimal point three places to the left, we can change the grams back to milligrams by moving the decimal point _____ places to the _____.

**14**

three
right

**14**

Let's see if you can complete a rule for changing grams to milligrams: To change grams to milligrams, move the decimal point _____ places to the _____ .

**15**

(a) 100 mg.
(b) 340 mg.
(c) 2 mg.
(d) 250 mg.
(e) 15 mg.

**15**

Work the following problems according to the rule that you have written:

| | | |
|---|---|---|
| (a) | 0.1 Gm. = | _____ mg. |
| (b) | 0.34 Gm. = | _____ mg. |
| (c) | 0.0020 Gm. = | _____ mg. |
| (d) | 0.25 Gm. = | _____ mg. |
| (e) | 0.015 Gm. = | _____ mg. |

**16**

500 mg.
2 capsules

**16**

The physician orders 0.5 Gm. of Panalba, and the label on the bottle reads 250 mg. per capsule. Since 0.5 Gm. is equal to _____ mg., you should give the patient _____ capsule(s).

**17**

4 tablets

**17**

Let's say that a physician orders 2 Gm. of Gantrisin as a "stat" dose and that the medication is dispensed in 500-mg. tablets. How many tablets should the patient receive? _____ .

**18**

(a) 500 mg.
(b) 5 mg.
(c) 0.03 Gm.
(d) 0.015 Gm.
(e) 0.004 Gm.
(f) 0.4 mg.
(g) 0.75 Gm.
(h) 600 mg.
(i) 0.3 Gm.
(j) 0.12 Gm.

To test your ability to change milligrams to grams, and grams to milligrams, complete the following table:

| | | | |
|---|---|---|---|
| (a) | 0.5 Gm. | _____ | mg. |
| (b) | 0.005 Gm. | _____ | mg. |
| (c) | 30 mg. | _____ | Gm. |
| (d) | 15 mg. | _____ | Gm. |
| (e) | 4 mg. | _____ | Gm. |
| (f) | 0.0004 Gm. | _____ | mg. |
| (g) | 750 mg. | _____ | Gm. |
| (h) | 0.6 Gm. | _____ | mg. |
| (i) | 300 mg. | _____ | Gm. |
| (j) | 120 mg. | _____ | Gm. |

# Post-test on the Metric System

A. Complete the following table of equivalents:

1. _____ ml. = 1 liter
2. _____ cc. = 1 ml.
3. _____ mg. = 1 gram

B. Write the correct abbreviations for the following:

4. Liter _____
5. Gram _____
6. Milliliter _____
7. Milligram _____
8. Cubic centimeter _____
9. Microgram _____

C. Write the following amounts as they would be read aloud:

10. 0.35 mg. _____
11. 0.2 mg. _____
12. 1.75 mg. _____
13. 0.5 Gm. _____
14. 0.6 ml. _____
15. 0.55 L. _____
16. 2.5 ml. _____
17. 0.04 mg. _____
18. 4.8 L _____
19. 7.5 Gm. _____
20. 10 mcg. _____

D. **Chart the following dosages, using the correct abbreviations and numbers:**

21. One and one-half grams       _____
22. Three-tenths milligram       _____
23. Seven-hundredths milliliter       _____
24. Three-fourths liter       _____
25. Two and one-half milligrams    _____

E. **Situations:**

26. A physician wishes to replace 2 liters of fluid lost by vomiting and diarrhea. If a bottle of intravenous fluids contains 1000 ml., how many bottles should the patient receive to replace the fluids lost?_____.
27. You must give a patient 0.015 Gm. of a certain drug, and the drug is dispensed in tablets of 5 mg. each. How many tablets would you give him?_____.
28. The proposed daily dosage for a medication is 2.4 Gm. The drug is available in 400 mg. tablets. How many tablets would be needed for a one-day supply?_____.
29. Suppose that a physician orders 100 mg. of a certain drug and the label on the bottle reads 0.1 Gm. per tablet. How many tablets would the patient receive? _____.
30. A child on pediatrics is given a 2.5 ml. dropperful of Erythrocin drops four times daily. He is receiving _____ cc. medication daily. If each 2.5 ml. contains 100 mg. of medication, he receives_____ Gm. of the drug daily.
31. A certain medication is available in 400 mg. tablets and a physician orders 2 Gm. per day. How many tablets would the patient receive each day?_____.

32. Mrs. Jamison is to receive 500 mg. of Thiosulfil Forte four times a day for treatment of cystitis. The only tablets available are scored tablets labeled 0.25 Gm. To supply the dosage of 500 mg. the patient should receive _____ tablet(s).

33. An elderly patient with prostatic cancer is to receive 1.25 mg. of Premarin three times daily. Because of difficulty in swallowing, he is receiving the liquid preparation. If 4 cc. contain 0.625 mg. he should receive _____ cc. for each dose. The liquid is supplied in 4-ounce (120cc.) bottles. This would be sufficient for _____ day(s).

34. Tybamate is a major tranquilizer. The physician has ordered 0.25 Gm. every four hours and you have available capsules containing 125 mg. each. How many capsules should the patient receive every four hours? _____.

35. The doctor has ordered 0.2 Gm. of Mebaral. You have available tablets of 32, 50, 100, and 200 mg. each. Which strength would be most appropriate to give and how many tablets would you give? _____.

# PART FIVE

# EXCHANGING UNITS OF WEIGHT AND MEASURE BETWEEN THE APOTHECARIES' AND THE METRIC SYSTEMS

# UNIT I

# Exchanging Units of Measure

*1*

metric

**1**

When you prepare to give a medication to a patient, you often find that a physician has ordered the drug in a unit of measure from the apothecaries' system, but that the drug has been prepared and is dispensed in a unit of measure from the metric system.

In this situation you must know both systems so that you can take the unit of measure from the apothecaries' system and find its approximate equivalent in the _____ system.

**2**

conversion

**2**

When you take an order in one system and find its approximate equivalent in another system, you are *converting*. The exchanging of units of weight and measure from one system to another is called _____.

**3**

cannot

**3**

In converting we find *approximately* the same weight or measure in a different system. We · can/cannot · say that the measurements are exactly the same.

**4**

1000 ml.

**4**

Let's consider how you would use conversion in preparing large amounts of solutions for various treatments.

You will recall that there are 1000 ml. in 1 liter. A quart in the apothecaries' system is equal to approximately 1 liter in the metric system. Therefore, there are approximately _____ ml. in 1 quart.

**5**

1 liter

**5**

Suppose that a physician orders 1 quart of soapsuds solution to be given as an enema, but that the only available container is a vessel graduated in liters. In measuring 1 quart of soapsuds solution in this container, you would prepare _____ liter(s).

**6**

500 cc.

**6**

There are 2 pints in 1 quart. Since a milliliter is the same amount as a cubic centimeter, you would calculate that there are approximately _____ cc. in 1 pint.

**7**

**7**

Let's say you must prepare a one-day supply of boric acid solution to be used for compresses. There are 8 patients receiving these compresses, and each

| | |
|---|---|
| 1 gallon | patient will need 500 ml. You know that you must prepare _____ gallon(s) of boric acid solution. |
| | If you worked that problem in Frame 7 correctly, go on to Frame 11. If you did not understand how to solve this problem, go on to Frame 8. |
| **8**<br>4000 ml. | **8**<br>Your first step in solving the problem would be to determine the total number of milliliters needed. Eight patients using 500 ml. each would require a total of _____ ml. |
| **9**<br>4 quarts | **9**<br>You would need 4000 ml. of the boric acid solution. If 1000 ml. equal approximately 1 quart, then 4000 ml. would be approximately the same as _____ quart(s). |
| **10**<br>1 gallon | **10**<br>Since there are 4 quarts in 1 gallon, and 4000 ml. are equal to 4 quarts, the amount needed for the boric acid compresses would be _____ gallon(s). |
| **11** | **11**<br>In another situation, you must prepare a supply of solution for 10 irrigations. |

1/2 gallon

You will need 200 ml. for each irrigation. The total amount of solution needed would be _____ gallon(s).

**12**

60 ml. (or cc.)

**12**

Sometimes it is necessary to convert ounces to milliliters. One ounce is equal to approximately 30 ml. A patient receiving milk and cream ℥ ii every hour would be given _____ ml. (or cc.) every hour.

**13**

45 ml. (cc.)

**13**

If a physician orders a dose of ℥ iss. of a certain medication, you could measure this in milliliters. You would give _____ ml. (cc.) of the medication to the patient.

**14**

240 cc.

**14**

If you were measuring and recording a patient's fluid intake in cubic centimeters, how many cc. would you record after a patient drinks an eight-ounce glass of water? _____.

**15**

15 ml.

**15**

Sometimes a physician will order Gelusil ℥ ss. You would give the patient _____ ml.

**16**

120 cc.
4 oz.

**16**

Suppose that a physician orders 4 cc. of elixir of phenobarbital every 4 hours for 30 doses, and you need to know how many fluid ounces to order from the pharmacy in order to have a sufficient amount of medication on hand.

Four cubic centimeters for 30 doses would be a total of _____ cc., or _____ ounce(s).

**17**

8 oz.

**17**

If a physician orders 12 cc. of a certain medication to be given 4 times a day for 20 doses, you must order a total of _____ fluid ounces from the pharmacy.

**18**

4 cc.

**18**

One dram in the apothecaries' system is equal to approximately 4 ml. in the metric system. If this is true, then 1 dram would contain approximately _____ cc.

**19**

8 ml.

**19**

If a physician orders ℥ ii of a medication, this would be approximately equivalent to _____ ml.

## 20

(a) 1 dr.
(b) 3 dr.
(c) 4 dr.
(d) 2 1/2 dr.

## 20

Just for practice, write the equivalents of the following amounts:

(a) 4 ml. _____ dr.
(b) 12 ml. _____ dr.
(c) 16 ml. _____ dr.
(d) 10 ml. _____ dr.

## 21

30 minims

## 21

It is often necessary to convert milliliters (or cubic centimeters) to minims, especially when preparing solutions to be given by injection. Therefore, it is important to remember that 1 ml. is equal to approximately 15 minims.

A 2-cc. syringe contains _____ minims.

## 22

10 minims

## 22

Let's say that you have dissolved a hypodermic tablet in 1 ml. of sterile water, and have calculated that you must give the patient only 2/3 of this amount. The patient will receive _____ minims of the solution.

## 23

75 mg.

## 23

Suppose that you have taken a 2-cc. ampule of Demerol from a container labeled 50 mg. per cc. If you gave a patient 22.5 minims, he would receive _____ mg. of the drug.

If you calculated the answer to the problem in Frame 23 correctly, go on to Frame 26. If you would like to see how this problem is solved, go on to Frame 24.

**24**

15 minims

**24**

To solve the problem, we must first realize that 50 mg. per cc. is the same as 50 mg. per 15 minims, because there are approximately _____ minims in 1 cc.

**25**

75 mg.

**25**

The patient received 22.5 minims, or 1.5 cc. If 1 cc. contains 50 mg., then 1.5 cc. would contain _____ mg.

**26**

10

**26**

Let's suppose that you have a 5-cc. vial of a drug and that the patient is to receive 7.5 minims daily. By dividing the total number of minims by the number of minims in each dose, you can determine the total number of doses in the vial. A 5-cc. vial of the drug will provide a patient with _____ daily doses of 7.5 minims each.

## 27

(a) 1 qt. = 1 L.
(b) 1 qt. =
    1000 ml.
(c) 1 pt. =
    500 ml.
(d) 1 oz. =
    30 ml.
(e) 1 dr. = 4 ml.
(f) 15 minims =
    1 ml.

## 27

In the process of converting, you must exchange measures in one system into approximate equivalents in another system. Test yourself and see how well you have learned the more commonly used equivalents.

| | Apothecaries' | | Metric |
|---|---|---|---|
| (a) | 1 quart | = _____ | liter(s) |
| (b) | 1 quart | = _____ | ml. |
| (c) | 1 pint | = _____ | ml. |
| (d) | 1 ounce | = _____ | ml. |
| (e) | 1 dram | = _____ | ml. |
| (f) | 15 minims | = _____ | ml. |

# Exchanging Units of Weight

**1**

proportion

**1**

Up to this point all the units we have used for conversion have been units of liquid measure. Now we are ready to convert units of weight. The simplest and most practical method for doing this is by using ratio and proportion. This method will stand you in good stead in computation of dosage too, and does not involve memorizing rules and formulas.

When confronted with the task of exchanging units of weight from one system of measure for another, you need not recall an extensive list of rules and formulas; you can use the simple method of ratio and _____.

**2**

1 and 15

**2**

You will remember that a ratio indicates the relationship between two quantities or two numbers. If you write 1:15, you are showing the relationship between _____ and _____ .

**3**

**3**

Setting up a ratio is simply a way of making a comparison between two quantities or numbers. The ratio of 1:15

means that one part of a given substance or thing is being compared to 15 parts of another substance or thing. An accepted equivalent for grains and grams is 1 Gm. = 15 gr. The ratio of 1 Gm. : 15 gr. means that _____ gram is comparable or equal to _____ grains.

1,
15

**4**

ratio

**4**

We can see, then, that the accepted equivalent of 1 Gm. = 15 gr. can be written as the ratio 1 Gm. : 15 gr. When you use an accepted equivalent from a table of equivalents, you can always express the equivalent as a _____.

**5**

Gm.,
gr.

**5**

In converting from one system to another it is very important to label the terms in a ratio. For example, 1:15 tells you nothing about the units of measure being represented. You must write the equivalent 1 Gram is equal to 15 grains as 1_____ :15 _____.

**6**

1/15

**6**

A ratio may be written as a fraction. The first term in the ratio is the numerator of the fraction and the second term is the denominator. The ratio 1 : 15 can be written _____.

(fraction)

**7**

the same value
   as

**7**

Since a ratio can be written as a common fraction, we can multiply or divide both terms of a ratio by the same number, just as we can multiply or divide both terms of a common fraction by the same number. This does not alter the value of the fraction or the ratio.

The ratio 2 Gm. : 30 gr. has · the same value as/twice the value of · the ratio 1 Gm.: 15 gr.

**8**

30 grains

**8**

A proportion shows equality between two ratios. We know that the ratio 1 Gm. : 15 gr. is the same as, or equal to, the ratio 2 Gm. : 30 gr. To express this equality, we write the proportion as 1 Gm. : 15 gr. = 2 Gm. : 30 gr. We can read this proportion to mean that 1 Gm. is comparable to 15 gr. in the same way that 2 Gm. are comparable to _____ _____.

**9**

2 Gm. : 30 gr.

**9**

A proportion is a quick way of showing the similarity between numbers of quantities. If we say "1 gram is similar to 15 grains in the same way that 2 grams are similar to 30 grains," we can see that the equality is expressed in the proportion: 1 Gm. : 15 gr. = _____ Gm.:_____ gr.

**10**

1 and 30
15 and 2

**10**

Each of the four parts of a proportion is called a term. The first and fourth are called the extremes; the second and third are called the means. In the proportion 1 Gm. : 15 gr. = 2 Gm. : 30 gr., the *extremes* are the numbers_____ and _____. The *means* are the numbers _____ and _____.

**11**

multiply

**11**

In a proportion the product of the means must always equal the product of the extremes. (In mathematics the word product indicates the result of multiplication.) To determine the product of the means and the product of the extremes, we must _____ 2 by 15 and 1 by 30.

**12**

extremes
means
 (either order)

**12**

Now our proportion of 1 Gm. : 15 gr. = 2 Gm. : 30 gr. becomes 30 = 30. A true proportion must always show that the product of the _____ is equal to the product of the _____ .

**13**

**13**

When one term of a proportion is not known, it is possible to find the value of this term. First we write our proportion and substitute X for the unknown term. Let's say that we have 1 Gm. : 15 gr. = X

Gm. : 3 gr. This proportion means that 1 gram is similar to 15 grains in the same way that _____ number of grams is similar to 3 grains.

X

**14**

**14**

$1 \times 3 = 3$

The proportion is 1 Gm. : 15 gr. = X Gm. : 3 gr. When we multiply the means we have 15 times X or 15X. When we multiply the extremes we have _____ X _____ which equals _____ .

**15**

**15**

X = 0.2 Gm.

Setting the product of the means equal to the product of the extremes, we have 15X = 3. We can determine the value of X by dividing 3 by 15. The value of X is

_____ .

**16**

**16**

left

These are the steps we have taken:

$$1 \text{ Gm. } : 15 \text{ gr. } = X \text{ Gm. } : 3 \text{ gr.}$$
$$15X = 3 \text{ (or } 3 \div 15)$$
$$X = 0.2 \text{ Gm.}$$

In the second step of evaluating X, the X must always be placed to the • left/right • of the equal sign.

**17**

**17**

A quick way to prove that your calculation of X is correct is to check to see whether the product of the means does

3
3

indeed equal the product of the extremes. If you calculated X as 0.2 Gm. in the proportion 1 Gm. : 15 gr. = X Gm. : 3 gr., you could determine that $15 \times 0.2$ = _____ and that $1 \times 3 =$ _____ .

## 18

grams to
grains

### 18

By now you must surely know that 1 gram is the approximate equivalent of 15 grains. Using this equivalent, try using ratio and proportion for some nursing problems involving converting grams to grains. Remember that in a proportion you must be careful that the units of measure are compared in the same order. If we compare grams to grains in the first ratio we must compare • grains to grams/grams to grains • in the second ratio.

## 19

7 1/2 gr.

### 19

We'll set up the first proportion for you.

$$1\,Gm. : 15\,gr. = 0.5\,Gm. : X\,gr.$$
$$1\,X = 15 \times 0.5$$
$$X = \underline{\hspace{1cm}} gr.$$

## 20

11 1/4 gr.
60 gr.
3 gr.
3 3/4 gr.

### 20

Here are some more for practice:

$$0.75\,Gm. = \underline{\hspace{1cm}} gr.$$
$$4\quad Gm. = \underline{\hspace{1cm}} gr.$$
$$0.2\quad Gm. = \underline{\hspace{1cm}} gr.$$
$$0.25\,Gm. = \underline{\hspace{1cm}} gr.$$

**21**

grains to
grams

**21**

Now we will suppose that the physician has ordered a drug in grains and it is dispensed in grams. Whenever you use conversion it is easier if you convert the unit of measure ordered to the unit of measure on hand. Since you must give medication from the units of measure you have available, it is more convenient in the above situation to convert · grains to grams/grams to grains ·

**22**

3.75 gr.

**22**

You need to convert gr. 3 3/4 to grams. Since the dosage on hand is measured in the metric system, and decimal numbers are used, the mixed number 3 3/4 should be changed to a decimal number. When setting up your proportion you should write gr. 3 3/4 as_____.

**23**

0.25 Gm.

**23**

Now you have the proportion:

1 Gm. : 15 gr. = X Gm. : 3.75 gr.
$$15 X = 3.75$$
$$X = \text{_____}$$

**24**

0.1 Gm.

**24**

Let's say that a physician orders Nembutal gr. iss, and that the drug is available in capsules labeled 0.1 Gm. each. Using ratio and proportion you will find that gr. iss is equal to_____Gm.

**25**

1 capsule

**25**

If the capsules are labeled 0.1 Gm. each and the physician has ordered gr. iss, it is obvious that the patient should receive _____ capsule(s).

**26**

0.8 Gm.
0.3 Gm.
3   Gm.
0.05 Gm.

**26**

Here are some practice problems:

12 gr. = _____ Gm.
 5 gr. = _____ Gm.
45 gr. = _____ Gm.
3/4 gr. = _____ Gm.

**27**

milligrams

**27**

In the above problems you have ex-changed grains and grams using the equivalent 1 Gm. = 15 gr. If you needed to exchange milligrams and grains you should use the equivalent 60 mg. = 1 gr. This can serve as your first ratio when converting _____ to grains.

**28**

30 mg. : X gr.

**28**

If, for instance, you needed to convert 30 mg. to an unknown number of grains, your proportion would be 60 mg. : 1 gr. = _____ : _____ .

**29**

**29**

Suppose that a physician orders 2 grains of a certain drug and that the dosage on hand is 60-mg. tablets. The first ratio is

60 mg. : 1 gr.
  = X mg. : 2 gr.

the conversion factor, 60 mg. = 1 grain. The proportion for converting is: _____ : _____ = _____ : _____ .

**30**

2 tablets

**30**

When you calculate the value of X, you find that the physician's order of 2 grains can be converted to 120 mg. If 1 tablet of the drug contains 60 mg., then _____ tablet(s) would contain 120 mg.

**31**

**31**

Suppose that a physician orders atropine gr. 1/150 and that the label on the bottle reads 0.2 mg. per tablet. You must know how many tablets to give the patient, but first you must convert the grains to milligrams.

0.4 mg.

After setting up your proportion and calculating X, you find that gr. 1/150 is equivalent to _____ mg.

**32**

2 tablets

**32**

Your problem was to determine how many tablets to give. You can again find the answer by using ratio and proportion:

0.2 mg. : 1 tablet = 0.4 mg. : X tablets
        X = _____ tablet(s)

**33**

60 mg. : 1 gr. =
   X mg. : 1/200
gr.

**33**

Suppose that a physician orders gr. 1/200 of scopolamine and that the drug is dispensed in 0.3-mg. tablets.

The proportion for converting the order into the dosage on hand is: _____ : _____ = _____ : _____.

**34**

1 tablet

**34**

When you calculate the value of X in this proportion, you find that 0.3 mg. is the equivalent of gr. 1/200. Now you know that the physician's order is the same as 0.3 mg. and that the patient should be given _____ tablet(s).

**35**

30 mg.

**35**

Suppose that a physician orders codeine gr. ss., and that the drug is dispensed in tablets of 15 mg. each.

After setting up your proportion and calculating the value of X, you find that gr. ss. is equivalent to approximately _____ mg.

**36**

2 tablets

**36**

Since you have found that the physician's order of gr. ss. is equivalent to approximately 30 mg., and since the drug is dispensed in tablets of 15 mg. each, you know that the patient should receive_____ tablet(s).

**37**

3/4 tablet

**37**

A physician orders gr. 1/4 of a certain drug, and the drug is dispensed in 20-mg. scored tablets. By using the ratio and proportion method, you can determine that the patient should receive _____ tablet(s).

**38**

1/20 gr.
1 tablet

**38**

In another situation, you find that a physician has ordered 3 mg. of a certain drug and that the dosage on hand is in gr. 1/20 tablets.

When you calculate the value of X, you find that 3 mg. are equal to _____ grain(s); therefore the patient should receive _____ tablet(s).

**39**

table

**39**

In working all the problems in this section you have used the equivalents 1 Gm. = 15 gr. and 60 mg. = 1 gr. These equivalents can be found in any table of accepted equivalents. Such a table usually is readily available in a hospital and should be used to avoid confusion and inaccuracy in calculation of dosage.

When a drug is ordered in one system and the dosage on hand is measured in another system, the safest and most accurate way to convert the dosage is by consulting a(n) _____ of accepted equivalents.

15 gr.
60 mg.

When the dosage ordered is not included in the table of equivalents, or a table is not available, you then use the equivalents you know and employ ratio and proportion to compute the dosage.

Two equivalents that you should be thoroughly familiar with at this point are 1 Gm. = _____ gr. and _____ mg. = 1 gr.

# Post-test on Exchanging Units of Weight and Measure

A. Complete the following table of equivalents:

1. 2 quarts = _____ liters
2. 1 gallon = _____ liters
3. 1/2 gallon = _____ ml.
4. 1000 ml. = _____ pints
5. 1 ounce = _____ ml.
6. 8 ml. = _____ drams
7. 2 ml. = _____ minims
8. 2/3 ml. = _____ minims
9. 20 minims = _____ ml.
10. 1/2 dram = _____ ml.
11. gr. 1/3 = _____ Gm.
12. gr. 7 1/2 = _____ Gm.
13. 0.25 Gm. = _____ grains
14. 2 Gm. = _____ grains
15. 0.2 Gm. = _____ grains

B. Situations:

16. Wet dressings of potassium permanganate 1:25,000 are to be applied 4 times daily. If 8 ounces of solution are necessary for each application, _____ L. will be needed for a 2-day supply.
17. An infant with anemia is given 20 minims of Feosol Elixir 3 times daily. This is a total of _____ ml. each day. If each 2 drams supplies 5 grains of medication, the infant is receiving _____ gr. daily.

18. A patient has been given 0.2 Gm. of a certain drug. This is approximately equivalent to _____ gr.

19. The doctor has ordered gr. vi. The tablets on hand are labeled 0.2 Gm. You should give _____ tablet(s).

20. A preoperative patient is receiving 180 grains of sulfasuxidine in 4 evenly divided doses. If each tablet contains 0.5 Gm., the patient is given _____ tablet(s) for each dose.

21. A physician orders gr. 1/6 of a certain drug. The dosage on hand is in 10-mg. tablets. The patient would receive _____ tablet(s).

22. The dosage desired is gr. 1/150. The drug on hand is in tablets of 0.2 mg. each. How many tablets would the patient receive? _____ .

23. The dosage desired is gr. 3/4. The drug on hand is in scored tablets of 15 mg. each. How many tablets would the patient receive? _____ .

24. A physician orders gr. 1/15 of a drug, and it is available only in 2-mg. tablets. You would give the patient _____ tablet(s).

25. The dosage desired is gr. 1/240 and the drug on hand is in 0.5-mg. scored tablets. The patient would receive _____ tablet(s).

# PART SIX

# PREPARING SOLUTIONS FOR PARENTERAL ADMINISTRATION

# UNIT I

# Powdered Drugs

solvent or
diluent

**1**

Some drugs are dispensed in powdered or crystalline form. A liquid such as sterile water or saline must be added to prepare these solid drugs for administration by injection. This liquid is called a solvent or a diluent.

The liquid used to prepare a solid drug for administration by injection is called a(n)_____ or a(n)_____ .

**2**

reconstitution

**2**

Most injectable powdered drugs are accompanied by printed information provided by the manufacturer and packaged with each vial. Specific directions for adding a liquid to the powdered drug are usually listed under the heading "Reconstitution."

When a liquid is added to the powdered drug in preparation for administration by injection, the procedure is referred to as _____ of the drug.

**3**

**3**

Reconstitution may be accomplished by adding sterile water or saline or some other liquid. Directions accompanying the vial usually specify the kind of solvent or diluent that should be used with a particular drug. When in doubt as to the type of liquid to use in reconstitution of a drug, this information can be obtained by reading the directions accompanying the _____ .

vial

**4**

**4**

amount

The directions for reconstitution of a drug usually tell precisely how much liquid must be added to obtain the desired dosage. The amount of liquid added has a direct bearing on the dosage of drug being administered.

When preparing a drug in powdered form for injection, one should look under the heading "Reconstitution" in the directions to determine the _____ of solvent or diluent to add.

**5**

**5**

0.5 ml.

For example, instructions for preparing a drug direct you to reconstitute the sterile dry powder by adding 1.5 ml. of sterile water. This provides a single dose of 2 ml. Since you added only 1.5 ml. of diluent, the volume of the dry drug would account for _____ ml. of finished solution.

**6**

displacement

**6**

Frame 5 gives an example of displacement. When drugs increase the volume of solution, one must read the manufacturer's directions, which will have taken into consideration the amount of _____ by the powdered drug after it has been dissolved.

**7**

2 ml.

**7**

Let's suppose that you must give 1 Gm. of Staphcillin. There is available a 6.0 Gm. vial with directions as follows: *Add 8.6 ml. of diluent (each ml. will contain 500 mg. Staphcillin).* After adding the diluent as directed, administer _____ ml. of the solution.

**8**

2.2 ml.

**8**

In another situation the patient is to receive 0.5 Gm. of Keflin. Directions accompanying the drug read as follows: *Each Gm. should be diluted with 4 ml. of sterile water for injection. This will provide 0.5 Gm. doses of 2.2 ml. each.*

After adding the diluent as directed withdraw _____ ml. of solution into the syringe in order to give the prescribed dose.

If you answered 2 ml. instead of 2.2 ml., you forgot about the powdered drug adding volume to the solution. Go back and reread Frames 5 and 6.

**9**

0.5 ml.

**9**

A patient is to receive 125 mg. of a certain drug. Directions for reconstitution read: *Add 1.2 ml. of sterile water; each 2 ml. will contain 0.5 Gm.*

After adding the diluent as directed, you will give the patient _____ ml. of the solution.

**10**

0.75 ml.

**10**

The physician has ordered 750 mg. of a certain drug. You have available a 10 Gm. multiple-dose vial. Directions for reconstitution read: *Add 8.5 ml. of sterile water. Each ml. will contain 1.0 Gm.* After adding the diluent as directed you will give _____ ml.

**11**

250 mg.

**11**

A patient is to receive 500 mg. of a certain drug. You have available 0.25 Gm. vials. Directions for reconstitution read: *Add 0.8 ml. of sterile water; each ml. will contain 0.25 Gm.*

After adding the diluent as directed, each ml. will contain _____ mg.

**12**

2 vials
2 ml.

**12**

In order to give the patient in Frame 11 a dosage of 500 mg., it will be necessary to reconstitute _____ vials and give the patient _____ ml.

diluent

When there are no directions accompanying powdered injectable drugs and there is no way of knowing how much volume the dry drug will add to the finished solution, one should consult a pharmacist for assistance in determining the amount of _____ to be added for a proper dosage.

# UNIT II

# Hypodermic Tablets

**1**

1 ml.

**1**

Hypodermic tablets are quite small and can easily be dissolved in sterile water or saline. The average amount of solution given by hypodermic injection is 1 ml.

When dissolving hypodermic tablets, the correct dosage of the drug will usually be dissolved in _____ of diluent.

**2**

3 ml.

**2**

Let's say that a physician orders atropine gr. 1/300, and that the dosage is available only in hypodermic tablets of gr. 1/100 each. If each milliliter of the solution is to contain gr. 1/300, you should dissolve the tablet in _____ ml. of sterile water.

If you answered the question in Frame 2 correctly, go on to Frame 6. If you missed this question, go on to Frame 3.

**3**

**3**

Let's stop and review the information given. First, we know that every 1 ml. of finished solution should contain gr. 1/300, because that is the amount of drug ordered by the physician, and the

average amount of solution given hypodermically is 1 ml. Now you set up your
first ratio as:

1/300 gr.:1 ml.

_____ gr. : _____ ml.

**4**

**4**

1/100 gr. : X ml.

When you set up the second ratio, you
find that you do not know the number
of milliliters to use as a diluent. You do
know, however, the number of grains in
each tablet on hand: each tablet contains
1/100 grains. The second ratio is written:

_____ gr. : _____ ml.

**5**

**5**

3 ml.

Now you have:

1/300 gr. : 1 ml. = 1/100 gr. : X ml.

When you solve this for X, you find that
the tablet should be dissolved in _____
ml. of diluent.

**6**

**6**

1/300 gr.

If you dissolve gr. 1/100 in 3 ml. and
give a 1 ml. injection, you are giving the
patient 1/3 of gr. 1/100, which equals
_____ grain(s) of the drug.
(fraction)

**7**

**7**

Suppose that a physician orders gr.
1/150 and the drug is dispensed in

tablets of 1/100 grains each. If 1 ml. is to contain gr. 1/150, you should dissolve 1 tablet of gr. 1/100 in_____ ml. of diluent and discard_____ ml. of finished solution.

1.5 ml.
0.5 ml.

**8**

**8**

2 or more

Sometimes the dosage ordered by a physician is larger than the amount contained in a single hypodermic tablet. When you convert the order into the dosage on hand and find that 1 tablet is not sufficient, you must use_____or more tablets, depending on the amount of drug needed.

**9**

**9**

3 tablets
90 mg.

It is easy to determine the number of tablets needed if we simply look at the dosage ordered and the amount on hand. For example, we cannot obtain 45 mg. of a drug from a single 30-mg. tablet. Therefore we must take the dosage from 2 tablets, or 60 mg.

If we need 75 mg. of a drug, and we have on hand only 30-mg. tablets, it will be necessary to use_____ tablet(s), which add up to_____ mg.

**10**

**10**

Your problem is to give 75 mg. in 1 ml. (15 minims). You have 90 mg. on hand (3, 30-mg. tablets). To give the patient

18
3
15

75 mg. of the drug you should dissolve the 3 tablets in _____ minims of diluent, discard _____ minims and give the patient _____ minims.

**11**

60 mg.

**11**

Suppose that you are instructed to give 50 mg. of a drug hypodermically, and the drug is available in 30-mg. tablets. To obtain 50 mg. in 15 minims of finished solution, you must use 2 tablets of 30 mg. each. Your proportion would be:

50 mg. : 15 minims = _____ mg. : X minims

**12**

18 minims
 3 minims
15 minims

**12**

Your proportion is:

50 mg. : 15 minims = 60 mg. : X minims

If 15 minims is to contain 50 mg. of the drug, you must dissolve 2 of the 30-mg. tablets in _____ minims of diluent, discard _____ m. and give the patient _____ m.

**13**

2 tablets
20 minims

**13**

Suppose that another physician's order reads scopolamine gr. 1/200, and you have on hand gr. 1/300 tablets. To obtain the dosage of gr. 1/200 in 15 minims of finished solution, you must dissolve _____ tablet(s) in _____ minims of diluent.

5 minims

When you have dissolved 2 of the gr. 1/300 tablets in 20 minims of diluent, and you are supposed to give 15 minims, you must discard _____ minims before giving the injection.

# UNIT III

## Stock Solutions

**1**

50 mg. : 1 ml.

**1**

In some instances, the drug on hand is already in solution and the amount of drug per milliliter is written on the label of the vial. A label reading "50 mg. per ml." tells you that the ratio of milligrams to milliliters is _____ : _____ .

**2**

35 mg. : X ml.

**2**

Since the drug is already in solution, you do not need to determine the amount of diluent to use. The unknown factor is the amount of solution to be given so that the correct dosage is obtained. The label on the vial gives us our first ratio.

Our second ratio shows the amount of drug ordered by the physician compared to the amount to be given in milliliters. If the physician orders 35 mg., our second ratio would be _____ mg. : _____ ml.

**3**

**3**

If a physician orders 35 mg. of Demerol and the label on the multiple-dose vial reads 50 mg. per ml., the proportion is written:

50 mg. : 1 ml. = 35 mg. : X ml.

The amount of solution to be given is _____ .

0.7 ml.

**4**

10.5 minims

**4**

Some syringes are calibrated in minims rather than tenths of a milliliter. To give the patient 0.7 ml. (or 0.7 of 15 minims), you should pull the plunger of the syringe back to the line marked _____ minims.

Arithmetically, the correct answer to the question in Frame 4 is 10.5 minims, but a minim is such a small amount that the number 10.5 should be rounded off to 11.

**5**

1.5 cc.

**5**

You are instructed to give 37.5 mg. of Leritine. The label on the 2-cc. ampule reads 50 mg. The patient should be given _____ cc. of the drug.

If you had no trouble finding the correct answer to the problem in Frame 5, go on to Frame 7. If you did not get the right answer, go on to Frame 6.

**6**

**6**

You probably missed the problem because you failed to notice that the ratio of drug to solution was 50 mg. : 2 cc., rather than 50 mg. : 1 cc.

Be very careful when you are reading labels on medication!

Your proportion should be:

50 mg. : 2 cc. = 37.5 mg. : X cc.

When you solve for X, you find that the patient should receive _____ cc.

1.5 cc.

**7**

20 minims

**7**

Let's say that you have a 2-cc. ampule of caffeine sodium benzoate, and that the ampule contains gr. viiss. If the physician orders gr. v, you should give the patient _____ minims.

Surely you didn't miss this one! If you did, go back and look at the question again. We asked for the number of minims to be given.

**8**

10 minims

**8**

Suppose that a physician orders gr. 1/6 of morphine sulfate. The drug is available in a multiple-dose vial labeled 15 mg. per cc. How many minims should the patient receive? _____.

If you did not have the correct answer to the problem in Frame 8, go on to Frame 9. If you were right, go on to Frame 11.

**9**

**9**

You seem to be forgetting that you must convert when a drug is ordered in one system and the supply on hand is in another system. We convert the dosage ordered by the physician into the units of the dosage on hand.

To determine the equivalent in milligrams for 1/6 grain, you write the proportion:

60 mg. : 1 gr. = X mg. : 1/6 gr.

When you solve for X, you find that 1/6 grain = _____ mg.

10 mg.

## 10

10

10 minims

The physician ordered 10 mg. and the dosage on hand is 15 mg. per cc. To determine the number of minims to be given the patient, you must change the cubic centimeters to minims. If 1 cc. = 15 minims, your proportion is:

15 mg. : 15 minims = 10 mg. : X minims

When you solve for X, you find that the patient should receive _____ minims.

## 11

11

15 minims

Suppose that a physician orders atropine 0.4 mg. The drug is available in a multiple-dose vial labeled gr. 1/150 per cc. You should give the patient _____ minims of atropine.

**12**

3 minims

**12**

Let's say that you have been instructed to give a patient 0.25 mg. of Serpasil. The drug is dispensed in 2-cc. ampules containing 2.5 mg. The patient should receive _____ minims of the drug.

**13**

0.24 cc. or 3.6 or 4 minims

**13**

The physician has ordered 6 mg. of Phenergan. The drug is available in an ampule labeled 25 mg. per cc. The patient should receive _____ cc. or _____ minims.

**14**

0.18 cc.

**14**

An order reads Atropine 0.15 mg. The label on the ampule reads 0.4 mg. per 0.5 cc. The patient should receive _____ cc.

**15**

0.75 cc.

**15**

The physician orders 750 mcg. of Vitamin $B_{12}$. The drug is available in a 10 cc. multiple-dose vial which is labeled 1000 mcg. per cc. The patient should receive _____ cc.

**16**

0.4 cc.

**16**

The order reads Reserpine 1 mg. The label on the container reads 5 mg. per 2 cc. The patient should receive _____ cc.

**17**

0.1 cc.

**17**

The order reads 0.25 mg. of Reserpine. The drug is available in an ampule labeled 5 mg. per 2 cc. The patient should receive _____ cc.

**18**

0.6 cc.

**18**

A physician orders liver extract 12 mcg. The label on the container reads 20 mcg. per cc. The patient should receive _____ cc.

**19**

0.4 cc.

**19**

An order reads Demerol 20 mg. The vial is labeled 25 mg. per 0.5 cc. The patient should receive _____ cc.

**20**

0.3 cc.

**20**

The order reads Hydrocortisone 8 mg. The multidose vial is labeled 25 mg. per cc. The patient should receive _____ cc.

# UNIT IV

# Drugs Measured in Units

*1*

cannot

**1**

Most drugs are standardized. This means that their active ingredients can be separated and chemically analyzed. Since the active chemical ingredients of these drugs are known, they can be measured according to the standard systems of measurement.

There are some drugs, however, that cannot be analyzed chemically. Since we cannot separate the active ingredients of these drugs, they · can/cannot · be measured according to the usual systems of measurement.

**2**

units

**2**

Drugs that cannot be analyzed by chemical means are standardized according to their effect on laboratory animals. These drugs are labeled in *units.* The word *"unit"* in this sense means the amount needed to bring about the desired effect in a laboratory animal. The strength of hormones, vitamins, and some other drugs must be determined by their effects on laboratory animals. These medications are labeled in _____ .

**3**

standards

**3**

All drugs must meet certain standards. When we see the words "U.S.P. Units" on a label, this means that the drug meets the _____ set by the United States Pharmacopeia.

**4**

diluent

**4**

Drugs that are labeled in units may be in solid or liquid form. If a drug comes in solid form, one must read the directions on the accompanying circular provided by the manufacturer to determine the amount of diluent to add to obtain correct dosage.

When a solid drug is measured in units, one must read the accompanying directions to find the amount of · diluent/ units · needed.

**5**

solution

**5**

Sometimes drugs that are labeled in units are already in solution when dispensed from the pharmacy. Since a diluent does not need to be added, you set up a proportion for the purpose of determining the amount of solution to be given.

When a drug is already in solution, we use ratio and proportion to determine the amount of _____ to be given so that the desired dosage is obtained.

## 6

units : ml.

## 6

The procedure for setting up the proportion for drugs already in solution is the same whether the drug is measured in grams or labeled in units. If the drug is labeled in grams, the ratio will be Gm: ml. If the drug is labeled in units, the first ration will be: _____ : _____.

## 7

40 units : 1 ml.
  = 50 units : X
ml.

## 7

The first ratio represents the dosage on hand and is expressed units : ml. The second ratio represents dosage ordered in units : amount of solution to be given.

Let's suppose that you have on hand a vial containing 40 units per ml., and a physician orders 50 units. The proportion would be:

_____ : _____ = _____ : _____ .

## 8

1.25 ml.

## 8

Your proportion is 40 units : 1 ml. = 50 units: X ml. When you solve for X, you find that the patient should receive _____ of the solution.

## 9

12 minims

## 9

If a physician orders 8000 units of heparin and the dosage on hand is 10,000 units per cc., the patient should receive _____ minims.

**10**

**10**

9 minims

Let's say a physician orders 3000 units. The drug is dispensed in vials of 5000 units per ml. The patient should receive _____ minims.

**11**

**11**

1.3 cc.

If you were asked to give a patient 400,000 units of penicillin, and the drug was available only in a multiple-dose vial containing 300,000 units per cc., you would give the patient _____ cc. of the drug.

**12**

**12**

1.5 ml.

A physician orders 60 units of ACTH to be given I.M., and the dosage on hand is 40 units per ml. The amount that you would give the patient is _____ ml.

**13**

**13**

1.2 cc. or 18 minims

The order reads heparin 12,000 U. The vial is labeled 10,000 units per cc. The patient should receive _____ cc. or _____ minims.

**14**

**14**

0.7 cc. or 11 minims

You are to give 35,000 U. of a certain drug. The label reads 50,000 units per cc. The patient should receive _____ cc. or _____ minims.

1.6 cc.

The order reads adrenal cortex 80 units. The drug is labeled 50 units per ml. The patient should receive _____ cc.

# Preparation of Insulin Dosage

**1**

units

## 1

In the previous section, you learned that some drugs are measured in units rather than in milligrams, grains, or grams. Insulin, being a hormone, is an example of this type of drug. If you were asked to administer a dosage of insulin from a commercially prepared solution, you would expect the prescribed amount to be measured in · units/mgms. ·

**2**

cc.

## 2

Insulin is presently available in varying strengths, depending on the number of units in a given amount of solution. Just as some drugs are measured in milligrams per cc., the strength of insulin is determined by the number of units per

———— .

**3**

## 3

Although there are several strengths of insulin on the market at the present time, the American Diabetes Association has recommended that eventually only one strength will be available and all other strengths phased out. The reason for this is to avoid confusion and error in the administration of insulin. The recommended strength to be used exclusively in the future is U. 100 insulin. In preparations of this strength, each cc. of solution contains _____ units of insulin.

100

**4**

**4**

In a vial of U. 100 insulin, the strength of the insulin is 100 units per _____ .

cc.

**5**

**5**

Insulin is a medication that usually is self-administered by the diabetic patient after he has been instructed in the technique of preparing and administering his own injections. In order to eliminate the need for calculating the volume of solution to be administered, a specially designed syringe is used. This syringe is calibrated in units, as shown in the drawing (p. 150). The drawing shows a U. 100 syringe which is to be used only for the administration of U. 100 insulin.

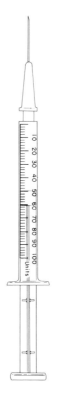

If a patient is to receive 60 units of U. 100 insulin, the plunger is pulled back and solution drawn up to the line designating · 60 units/60 cc. ·

60 units

**6**

**6**

The insulin syringe makes it possible to obtain a correct dosage without mathematical calculation or conversion from units to cc. It is very important, however, that only a syringe calibrated for U. 100 insulin be used to prepare and administer insulin that is labeled U. _____.

**7**

There are several kinds of insulin syringes designed for the administration of U. 100 insulin. The drawing below shows a syringe that may be used for insulin doses under 35 units.

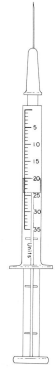

If the patient is to receive 30 units of insulin, using U. 100 insulin and the syringe pictured on page 151, the plunger would be pulled back and solution drawn up to the line designating _____ units.

30

**8**

label

**8**

You may wonder why we have spent so much time explaining something which is so very simple. It is obviously very easy to prepare a dosage of insulin when you have a solution labeled U. 100 and a syringe designed for the administration of insulin of that strength. Confusion arises, however, when there are available varying strengths of insulin and syringes which may be calibrated for differing strengths of insulin. That is why you are urged to be sure that the syringe you are using is designed for the strength of insulin you have on hand. The most reliable source of information regarding the strength of insulin being used is the _____ on the vial.

9

**9**

Until there is only one strength of insulin available, you may have to contend with preparing insulin that is labeled U.20, U.40, or U.80. You remember that the label U.100 tells you that there are 100 units per cc. of solution in

40

the vial. The term U.40 tells you that there are _____ units of insulin per cc. of solution.

**10**

## 10

cc.

A vial of insulin labeled U.80 is one in which there are 80 units in each _____ of solution.

**11**

## 11

U.40

Just as there are syringes designed for U.100 insulin, there also are syringes designed for U.40 and U.80 insulin. Hopefully these will soon become obsolete and will no longer be available as a source of confusion in the administration of insulin. Until that time arrives, however, you should be familiar with these varying strengths of insulin, particularly in your dealings with older persons who are familiar with U.40 and U.80 insulin and are not willing or are unable to discard their old ways of doing things.

The drawing shows one syringe calibrated for both U.40 and U.80 insulin.

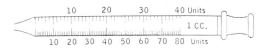

If you are to give 30 units of U.40 insulin, you would read the side of the scale calibrated for · U.40/U.80 · insulin.

**12**

U.80

**12**

Using the same type of insulin syringe pictured above, if you are to give 40 units of U.80 insulin, you would read the side of the syringe calibrated for · U.40/U.80 · insulin.

**13**

40

**13**

If you wish to give 40 units of insulin and you are using U.80 strength, you should read the side calibrated for U.80 insulin and draw up the solution to the line indicating _____ units.

**14**

40

**14**

Look at the drawing again and locate the line indicating 20 units on the U.40 scale. The corresponding line on the U.80 scale reads _____ units.

**15**

**15**

It should now be apparent that extreme caution must be exercised in the administration of varying strengths of insulin. In order to avoid error it is imperative that the label on the vial of insulin be read to determine its strength and that the syringe be examined to determine the strength of insulin for which it is designed.

should not

If you are giving insulin from a vial labeled U.100, you · should/should not · use a syringe calibrated for U.40 and U.80 insulin.

---

**16**

0.5

**16**

In the future, U.100 insulin will be the only strength available because it lends itself very readily to calibrations in the metric system. If, for example, there were no syringes specifically calibrated for the administration of a dosage of U.100 insulin, and the patient is to receive 50 units, you could use a 1-cc. or a 2-cc. syringe and give the patient _____ cc. of U.100 insulin.

---

**17**

50

**17**

You know that 0.5 cc. of U.100 insulin would provide 50 units of insulin because 0.5 of 100 is _____.

---

**18**

0.75 or 3/4

**18**

Let's say that you wish to give 75 units of U.100 insulin, but a syringe calibrated in units is not available. Using a 1-cc. or a 2-cc. syringe, you would give the patient _____ cc. of U.100 insulin.

---

**19**

**19**

If it should ever become necessary to use U.40 or U.80 insulin and a 1-cc. or 2-cc.

syringe, you could use ratio and proportion to calculate the volume of solution to give. Although this eventuality is not likely to occur, there is no reason to become upset should it happen, as long as you remember the rules for calculation of dosages using other types of medications. You recall that the first ratio for the proportion is obtained from the label on the drug. If the vial is labeled U.40, then your first ratio would be _____ units : 1 cc.

40

**20**

1 cc.

**20**

The first ratio would be 40 units : 1 cc., because the term U.40 means that there are 40 units in each _____ of solution.

**21**

40 units : 1 cc. =
30 units : X cc.

**21**

The second ratio shows the relation between the dosage ordered and the unknown number of cc. (X) to be given.

If the physician orders 30 units of insulin and the drug on hand is U.40 insulin, the proportion is written _____

: _____ = _____ : _____ .

**22**

0.75 cc.

**22**

Solving for X, you find that the patient is to receive _____ cc. of U.40 insulin in order to obtain 30 units.

**23**

0.4 cc.

**23**

Suppose you needed to give 35 units of insulin and the drug is available as U.80 insulin. The patient should receive _____ cc.

**24**

U.80

**24**

You can see that using a 1-cc. or 2-cc. syringe is not the most accurate method for the administration of insulin. Whenever possible, it is best to use a syringe that is calibrated for the specific strength of insulin on hand. If you are administering U.80 insulin, it would be most accurate to use a syringe calibrated for _____ insulin.

# Post-test on Preparing Solutions for Parenteral Administration

## A. Situations:

1. Directions accompanying an injectable powdered drug read as follows: *Add 1.7 ml. of diluent (each ml. will contain 500 mg.).* In order to give 0.5 Gm. of the drug, give _____ ml. of the solution.

2. You must give 0.25 Gm. of an antibiotic. Directions accompanying the drug read: *Add 8.6 ml. of diluent (each ml. contains 500 mg.).* After adding the diluent, give the patient _____ ml. of the solution.

3. The dosage on hand is a hypodermic tablet of gr. 1/100. The dosage desired is gr. 1/150. How much diluent would be used to obtain the correct amount of drug in 1 ml.? _____.

4. The dosage desired is gr. 1/4. The hypodermic tablets on hand contain gr. 1/6 each. How many tablets would be used? _____. How much diluent would be used to obtain the correct dosage in one ml.? _____.

5. The physician orders 30 mg. of Demerol. The drug on hand is a vial labeled "50 mg. per cc." How many minims would be given to obtain the correct dosage? _____.

6. The dosage on hand is 50 mg. per 2 cc. The physician orders 37.5 mg. How many cc. of stock solution would you give the patient? _____.

7. The physician orders 0.8 mg. of Levo-Dromoran. The drug on hand is a vial labeled 2 mg. per cc. How many minims of solution would be given? _____.

8.  A physician orders gr. 1/300 of a certain drug. The dosage on hand is a hypodermic tablet of gr. 1/200 each. How much diluent would be used to dissolve the tablet so that the correct dosage is obtained in one ml.? _____ .

9.  The dosage ordered is 25 units of insulin. Using a 2-cc. or tuberculin syringe and a vial of U.100 insulin, you would give the patient _____ ml.

10. A physician orders 60 units of insulin and the strength on hand is U.80 insulin. In order to give an accurate dosage, you would need to use a syringe calibrated for _____ insulin.

# PART SEVEN

# RATE OF
# FLOW OF
# INTRAVENOUS
# FLUIDS

**1**

The monitoring of the rate of flow of intravenous fluids is a nursing responsibility. The rate of flow is measured in drops per minute. When a physician orders "2000 ml. $D_5W$ in 16 hours," it will be your responsibility to adjust the rate of flow so that the patient receives a total of 2000 ml. of $D_5W$ in _____ hours.

**2**

rate

**2**

Some companies which manufacture intravenous administration sets also provide a slide rule for determining the number of drops per minute that must be given to obtain the correct rate of flow over a period of hours. When such a slide rule is available, it can be used to determine the _____ of flow.

**3**

proportion

**3**

When such a slide rule is not available, it is necessary to use one's own resources to calculate the rate of flow in the same way that it is possible to calculate the dosage of medication when a table of equivalents is not available. It is possible, then, for you to compute the rate of flow for intravenous fluids by using ratio and _____ .

**4**

drops

**4**

One important factor in determining the rate of flow is the size of the drops of fluid being administered to the patient. Since you will be counting the drops, you will need to know something about the size of the _____ .

**5**

drops

**5**

The size of the drops determines the number of drops per milliliter. Intravenous sets vary in the size of the openings in the drip chamber and so these sets will vary in the size of the _____ passing through the chamber.

**6**

10

**6**

Packages for intravenous administration sets are labeled according to the number of drops per milliliter. For example, one type of set is labeled "10 drops per ml." This means that when using this type of set for administering intravenous fluids, one ml. is equal to _____ drops.

**7**

**7**

This information is used in the same way that one uses the information on a label of a vial of medication. You will recall that "50 mg. per ml." on a vial of medication is used as the first ratio in the proportion in setting it up to solve a

10 drops: 1 ml.

dosage problem. If the intravenous set package reads "10 drops per ml.," the first ratio should be _____ : _____ .

**8**

**8**

10 drops: 1 ml. = X drops: 1000 ml.

Let's suppose that a physician has ordered 1000 ml. of fluid by continuous intravenous drip to be given in 8 hours. The information on the intravenous set package reads "10 drops per ml." The first step in the problem is to determine the total number of drops in 1000 ml. The proportion should read

_____ : _____ = _____ : _____ .

**9**

**9**

10 drops: 1 ml.

If you got the correct answer, go on to Frame 11. If you did not set up the proportion correctly, it may be that you forgot the importance of the information on the intravenous set package. It read "10 drops per ml." Your first ratio is _____ : _____ .

**10**

**10**

You know that there are 10 drops per milliliter and you need to know the number of drops in 1000 ml. You then say to yourself, "My answer must be in drops . . . so if there are 10 drops in one milliliter, then how many drops (X) are in 1000 milliliters?" The proportion

10 drops: 1 ml. =
  X drops: 1000
  ml.

should read _____ : _____ =

_____ : _____ .

**11**

10,000

**11**

Having set up the proportion as 10 drops: 1 ml. = X drops: 1000 ml., and solving it for "X," you find that X = _____ drops.

**12**

minutes

**12**

You know now that the patient is to receive 10,000 drops. The physician has ordered the fluids to be given by continuous intravenous drip over a span of eight hours. It is unreasonable to think that monitoring the rate of flow would involve counting this many drops for eight hours. A good estimate of the rate of flow can be obtained by counting the number of drops per minute. Your next step, then, is to determine the number of _____ in eight hours.

**13**

480

**13**

Since there are 60 minutes in one hour, there are _____ minutes in eight hours.

**14**

10,000 drops:
  480 minutes

**14**

The patient is to receive 10,000 drops in 480 minutes. The first ratio in the next step in solving the problem is

_____ : _____ .

**15**

10,000 drops:
   480 minutes =
   X drops : 1
minute

**15**

You will be counting the number of drops in only one minute. Therefore, the proportion should be _____ : _____ = _____ : _____ .

**16**

20.8 or 21

**16**

In solving for "X" you find that the rate of flow should be _____ drops per minute.

**17**

10 drops : 1 ml.

**17**

A physician has ordered 2000 ml. of $D_5W$ to be given I.V. in 12 hours. The information on the package of the intravenous administration set reads "10 drops per milliliter." The first ratio should be _____ : _____ .

**18**

10 drops : 1 ml. =
   X drops : 2000
ml.

**18**

If you wrote the first ratio as 10 drops: 1 ml., you were correct. Now you must determine the total number of drops the patient is to receive. Your proportion should be _____ : _____ = _____ : _____ .

**19**

20,000
20,000

In solving the proportion 10 drops : 1 ml. = X drops : 2000 ml., you will find that X = _____ drops. Therefore, there are _____ drops in 2000 ml.

**20**

**20**

720

The patient is to receive 20,000 drops in 12 hours. Since there are 60 minutes in an hour, there are _____ minutes in 12 hours.

**21**

**21**

27.7 or 28

Now you know that the patient is to receive 20,000 drops in 720 minutes. In setting up the proportion and solving for "X," you find that the rate of flow should be _____ drops per minute.

**22**

**22**

milliliters

If your answer was correct, go on to Frame 27. If your answer was not correct, it may be that you are having difficulty setting up your proportion. Remember that you must always compare units of measure in the same order. If you compare drops to milliliters in one ratio, you must compare drops to _____ in the second ratio.

**23**

2000

**23**

You know that by using the regular intravenous administration set that there are 10 drops per milliliter. Now you need to know how many drops are in the total amount of fluid to be received by the patient. Your first step is to convert the milliliters to drops. The physician has ordered 2000 ml. of fluid. Therefore, the proportion should be 10 drops :1 ml. = X drops: _____ ml.

**24**

20,000

**24**

Using the proportion you have set up and solving for "X," you find that the answer is _____ drops.

**25**

720

**25**

The patient is to receive 20,000 drops in 12 hours. There are 60 minutes in one hour; therefore, there are _____ minutes in 12 hours.

**26**

27.7 or 28

**26**

The rate of flow is 20,000 drops in 720 minutes. You need to know how many drops the patient is to receive in one minute. The proportion is 20,000 gtt.: 720 min. = X gtt. : 1 min. 720X = 20,000; so X =_____ drops.

**27**

drops

**27**

Before going on to other examples of problems you may encounter when monitoring the rate of flow of intravenous fluids, it may be well to review the steps to be taken in solving the problems. The physician orders the total amount in milliliters, but you will be counting in drops. Your first step is to convert the total amount in milliliters to the total amount in _____ .

**28**

60

**28**

After finding the total number of drops to be given the patient, you must determine the total number of minutes in which the fluids are to be administered. Since there are 60 minutes in one hour, you can find the total number of minutes by multiplying the specific number of hours by _____ .

**29**

27.7 or 28

**29**

The steps are as follows:
   Step 1: Find total number of drops
   Step 2: Find total number of minutes
   Step 3: Find number of drops per minute

If the patient is to receive 20,000 drops in 720 minutes, the rate of flow can be determined by solving for "X."

20,000 gtt.: 720 min. = X gtt.: 1 min.

The answer is _____ drops per minute.

**30**

6000

---

**30**

In another situation, the physician has ordered 2 units (500 ml. each) of packed cells to be given in 8 hours. When reading the administration set package, you find that there are 6 drops per milliliter. Using this information, you calculate that the patient is to receive a total of _____ drops in 8 hours.

---

**31**

480

---

**31**

The patient will receive 6000 drops in 8 hours, or _____ minutes.

---

**32**

12.5 or 13

---

**32**

If the patient is to receive 6000 drops in 480 minutes, the rate of flow should be _____ drops per minute.

---

**33**

46.8 or 47

---

**33**

Suppose the physician orders 3000 ml. in 16 hours and the package for the intravenous administration set reads 15 drops per ml. The rate of flow should be _____ drops per minute.

---

**34**

62.5 or 63

---

**34**

In another situation, a pediatrician orders 500 ml. in 8 hours. The intravenous administration set package reads "60 drops per milliliter." The rate of flow should be _____ drops per minute.

**35**

41.6 or 42

**35**

A physician orders 4000 ml. of fluid to be given in 24 hours. The package directions read "15 drops per ml." The rate of flow should be _____ drops per minute.

**36**

41.6 or 42

**36**

A pediatrician orders 1000 ml. of fluid to be given in 24 hours. The intravenous administration set package states that there are 60 drops per milliliter. The rate of flow should be _____ drops per minute.

**37**

156.2 or 156
78.1 or 78

**37**

A severely burned patient is to receive a total amount of 10 liters of intravenous fluids in a 24-hour period. One-half of the total is to be given during the first 8 hours, and the remainder during the next 16-hour period. If the package of the intravenous administration set reads "15 drops per ml.," then _____ drops per minute would be given during the first 8 hours and _____ drops per minute during the next 16 hours.

**38**

**38**

The second post-burn day the patient is to receive half the total amount of intravenous fluids he received during the first 24-hour period. This amount is to

52

be evenly divided over 24 hours. The patient should receive _____ drops per minute.

**39**

15.6 or 16

**39**

The third post-burn day, intravenous fluids are restricted to a total of 1500 ml. in 24 hours. The rate of flow would be _____ drops per minute.

# Post-test

1. A patient is receiving packed cells at the rate of 1 liter per 8 hours. If the package of the blood administration set states "6 drops per ml.," the rate of flow is_____ drops per minute.

2. A patient returning from the Operating Room has 750 ml. of I.V. fluid remaining in the container. You are instructed by the physician to complete the remaining fluid in 2 hours. The administration set attached to the intravenous fluid is a regular set having 10 drops per milliliter. The rate of flow will be _____ drops per minute.

3. The physician has calculated that the patient should receive 2500 ml. of intravenous fluid every 24 hours. If you are using an intravenous administration set that has 15 drops per milliliter, then the rate of flow should be _____ drops per minute.

4. A child is to receive 250 ml. of packed cells in 4 hours. The I.V. administration set is calibrated so that there are 6 drops in one milliliter. The rate of flow should be _____ drops per minute.

5. A pediatric patient will be given 1500 ml. of fluid intravenously in 24 hours. There are 60 drops per ml. using the pediatric I.V. administration set. The child will receive _____ drops per minute.

# PART EIGHT

# PREPARING LARGE AMOUNTS OF SOLUTIONS

# Pure Drugs

**1**

liquid

**1**

Solutions may be prepared from pure drugs or from strong stock solutions. In this unit, we will be concerned only with pure drugs. When we speak of pure drugs, we mean unadulterated substances in solid or liquid form. Making a solution from a pure drug involves dissolving a solid substance, or diluting a _____ substance.

**2**

proportion

**2**

There are several different ways to determine the amount of pure drug to use in preparing a solution of a certain strength. Since you are familiar with ratio and proportion, we will use this method.

To prepare a solution from a pure drug, you may determine the amount of pure drug needed by finding the value of an unknown in a _____.

**3**

**3**

In a proportion, the letter X represents the unknown factor. When you are using a proportion to find the amount of pure drug needed to prepare a given amount

| | of finished solution, the X represents |
|pure drug| the amount of _____ _____ required. |

**4**

pure drug
finished
 solution

**4**

When you prepare a solution, you must first decide how much of the *finished* solution you will need. The first ratio of the proportion will show the amount of pure drug contained in this amount of *finished* solution.

The first ratio of the proportion will be: amount of _____ _____: known amount of_____ _____.

**5**

5:100

**5**

In addition to knowing the amount of finished solution you will need, you must also know the strength desired for this solution. This strength is the second ratio of the proportion.

Let's say that you will need a 5% solution. The term "5%" means that there will be 5 parts of a substance in every 100 parts of the whole solution. Expressed as a ratio, 5% is the same as:

_____ : _____

**6**

**6**

Now we can see that a proportion can be set up for a situation in which we need

X : 1000 =
5 : 100

to prepare 1000 ml. of a 5% solution. We will use the proportion to determine the amount of pure drug needed. The proportion will express, X parts of pure drug: _____ parts of finished solution = _____ parts: _____ parts.

**7**

grams

**7**

We know that we must use units of measure to express the parts or amounts needed for the solution and the pure drug. The gram and the milliliter are the acceptable equivalents for solids and liquids, respectively.

The finished solution will be measured in milliliters. The pure drug in liquid form will be measured in milliliters. The pure drug in solid form will be measured in

_____.

**8**

5 Gm. : 100 ml.

**8**

Now you may ask how we can compare grams to milliters in one ratio and then compare a percentage to 100 in the other ratio. Actually, the term "5% solution" means that there are to be 5 Gm. or 5 ml. of the pure drug in every 100 ml. of finished solution. A 5% solution made from a solid pure drug can be written as the ratio: _____ Gm. : _____ ml.

**9**

X Gm. : 2000
  ml = 2 Gm.
  : 100 ml.

**9**

Now let's see how we set up a proportion for another situation. Suppose that you must prepare 2000 ml. of a 2% solution using boric acid crystals.

Because the pure drug is a solid, the proportion will compare grams to milliliters and will be written: _____ : _____ = _____ : _____.

**10**

40 Gm.

**10**

You solve for X to find how much pure drug should be used in 2000 ml. so that there will be 2 Gm. in every 100 ml. Your proportion is X Gm. : 2000 ml. = 2 Gm. : 100 ml.

The amount of pure drug needed for 2000 ml. is _____ Gm.

**11**

X Gm. : 1000
  ml. = 2.5 Gm.
  : 100 ml.

**11**

Suppose that a physician orders compresses using a 2 1/2% solution of magnesium sulfate. You will need to prepare 1 quart of this solution. Your proportion for this would be: _____ : _____ = _____ : _____.

If you set up the correct proportion for the problem in Frame 11, go on to Frame 14. If you did not get the right proportion, go on to Frame 12.

**12**

metric
metric

**12**

Solutions may be ordered according to the apothecaries' system, but the _____ system is the one most often used for weighing and measuring drugs because of its accuracy. When a solution is ordered in the apothecaries' system, the amount of finished solution should be converted to the _____ system.

**13**

1000 ml.

**13**

Since the physician has ordered 1 quart of a 2 1/2% solution, we must convert 1 quart to _____ before setting up the proportion.

**14**

5 Gm.

**14**

In another situation, a physician orders warm saline gargles using a 1% solution. The amount of sodium chloride needed to prepare 1 pint of solution would be

_____.

**15**

5 Gm.

**15**

Another time, you find that you must prepare 2000 ml. of a 1/4% solution. The pure drug is in solid form.

After setting up your proportion and solving for X, you find that you will need _____ of pure drug.

**16**

X ml. : 4000 ml.
  = 2 ml. : 100
ml.

**16**

Cresol solution is frequently used as a disinfectant. The solution is prepared from a pure liquid drug. If you needed to prepare 1 gallon of a 2% solution of cresol, your proportion would be:

_____ : _____ = _____ : _____.

**17**

80 ml.

**17**

Solving for X, you find that to prepare 1 gallon of a 2% cresol solution you will need_____ml. of the pure drug.

**18**

X Gm. : 2000
  ml. = 1 Gm.
  : 1000 ml.

**18**

Sometimes the strength of a solution is ordered as a ratio, such as 1 : 1000. In this case, your second ratio is already set up for you. Let's say you needed 2000 ml. of a 1 : 1000 solution. Your proportion is written: _____ Gm.: _____ ml. = _____Gm.: _____ml.

**19**

2 Gm.

**19**

After solving for X, you find that to prepare 2000 ml. of a 1 : 1000 solution, you will need_____Gm. of pure drug.

**20**

40 ml.

**20**

Let's suppose that you must prepare 1 gallon of a 1 : 100 solution. The pure drug is available in liquid form. You would use _____of pure drug.

3960 ml.

**21**

When preparing solutions, the correct procedure is to put the pure drug in a graduated container and add to it enough of the diluent to produce the desired amount of finished solution.

In a previous situation, you used 40 ml. of pure drug to make a solution. The amount of diluent needed to make this a 4000-ml. finished solution would be _____ ml.

**22**

8 Gm.

**22**

To prepare 80 ml. of a 10% solution, one would need to use _____ of pure drug in solid form.

**23**

24 tablets

**23**

Let's say that you must make 0.4 liters of a 3% solution. You have on hand a pure drug in the form of 0.5 Gm. tablets. To prepare the solution, you would use _____ tablet(s).

If you answered the question in Frame 23 without difficulty, go on to Frame 26. If you did not completely understand how we got the answer, go on to Frame 24 for an explanation.

**24**

**24**

You will recall that a 3% solution means that there are 3 Gm. or 3 ml. of solute for every 100 ml. of finished solution. Since the second ratio of the proportion compares grams to milliliters, the first ratio must also compare grams to milliliters.

The correct ratio for X grams to 0.4 liters would be: X Gm. :_____ ml.

400 ml.

**25**

24 tablets

## 25

Your proportion is now X Gm. : 400 ml. = 3 Gm. : 100 ml. When you solve for X, you find that you will need 12 Gm. of the pure drug. To obtain 12 Gm. from the 0.5 Gm. tablets, you would need to use _____ tablet(s).

**26**

2 Gm.

## 26

Suppose that you wish to prepare 2000 ml. of a 1 : 1000 solution from 5 gr. tablets. Using the proportion X Gm. : 2000 ml. = 1 Gm. : 1000 ml., you find that you will need _____ Gm. of pure drug.

**27**

30 grains
6 tablets

## 27

In this problem, the pure drug was available in 5 gr. tablets. If you need 2 Gm., this would be the same as_____ grain(s) or _____ tablet(s).

**28**

1 tablet

## 28

To prepare 1 liter of a 1 : 2000 solution, using gr. viiss. tablets, one would have to use _____ tablet(s).

**29**

100 ml.
3900 ml.

**29**

Suppose that the pure drug on hand is a liquid, and that you need to prepare 4 liters of a 2 1/2% solution.

You would use _____ml. of pure drug and_____ml. of diluent.

**30**

36 Gm.

**30**

The strength of physiological saline (normal saline) is 0.9%. To prepare 1 gallon of normal saline using sodium chloride crystals, one would need_____Gm. of the pure drug.

**31**

1%

**31**

A 5% solution means that there are 5 parts of one substance in every 100 parts of the solution. If you used 10 Gm. of pure drug in 1000 ml. of finished solution, you would have 10 parts of pure drug in every 1000 parts of solution. This is a ratio of 10 : 1000, or 1 : 100. Expressed as a percentage, this would be _____%.

**32**

8%

**32**

Let's say that you have used 80 ml. of pure drug in 1000 ml. of solution. The ratio would be 80 : 1000. The percentage of your finished solution would be _____%.

# UNIT II

# Stock Solutions

**1**

stock

**1**

The preceding problems were concerned with the preparation of solutions from a pure drug. Sometimes, however, one must prepare solutions from a strong stock solution.

Hospitals keep on hand concentrated solutions from which various strengths of weaker solutions can be made. These strong solutions are called _____ solutions because they are always kept on hand.

**2**

less

**2**

We do not use the same proportion for stock solutions as for pure drugs. When we use a strong stock solution to make a weaker solution, we are dealing with two different strengths. The strength of the finished solution will be · less/greater · than the strength of the stock solution.

**3**

**3**

Our proportion for stock solutions compares amounts of the solutions as well as their strengths. The first ratio compares the lesser amount to the greater amount. The second ratio must follow the same

lesser
greater

order and compare the _____ strength to the _____ strength.

**4**

**4**

X ml. : 1000 ml. = 2% : 4%

Now we have our proportion for preparing a weaker solution from a strong stock solution. The lesser amount of stock solution is to the greater amount of stock solution as the lesser strength is to the greater strength.

If you need to prepare 1000 ml. of a 2% solution from a 4% stock solution, your proportion would be: X ml. : _____ ml. = _____% : _____%.

**5**

**5**

stock solution

Your proportion is set up to determine the amount of stock solution to use. It is written X ml. : 1000 ml. = 2% : 4%. You solve for X, and find that 500 ml. is the amount of _____ _____ to be used.

**6**

**6**

500 ml.

Your problem was to prepare 1000 ml. of finished solution. If you used 500 ml. of stock solution, the amount of diluent to be added would be _____.

**7**

**7**

Suppose that you needed to prepare 1 pint of a 2% solution from a 10% stock

X ml. : 500 ml
= 2% : 10%

solution. Your proportion for this would be: _____ : _____ = _____ : _____.

**8**

100 ml.
400 ml.

**8**

Your proportion is X ml. : 500 ml. = 2% : 10%. When you solve for X, you find that the amount of stock solution needed is _____ and the amount of diluent to be added is _____.

**9**

75 cc.
675 cc.

**9**

Let's say that you need 750 cc. of a 5% solution. The stock solution on hand is a 50% solution. To make 750 cc. of finished solution, pour _____ of stock solution into a graduated pitcher and add _____ of diluent.

**10**

1 part
1000 parts

**10**

The strength of a stock solution may be expressed by a percentage or by a ratio. Zephiran Chloride, for example, is available in strengths of 1 : 1000, 1 : 3000, and so forth.

A 1 : 1000 solution would have _____ part(s) of Zephiran Chloride in every _____ parts of finished solution.

**11**

**11**

When the strength of a stock solution is expressed in a ratio, it is necessary to

1/3000

change the ratio to a fraction before setting up the proportion. The ratio of 1 : 3000 can be written as the common fraction _____.

**12**

1/3000 : 1/1000

**12**

You know that the proportion for preparing a weaker solution from a stronger solution is lesser amount: greater amount = lesser strength : greater strength. If you were to prepare a 1 : 3000 solution from a 1 : 1000 solution, the second ratio would be set up as _____ : _____.

If you missed the proportion in Frame 12, you probably forgot that the larger the denominator of a fraction, the less the value of the fraction. Remember that 1/8 of a pie is a smaller slice than 1/4 of a pie.

**13**

X cc. : 500 cc. = 1/3000 : 1/1000

**13**

Now let's see how we would set up the entire proportion in a clinical situation. You must prepare 500 cc. of a 1 : 3000 solution, and the stock solution on hand is 1 : 1000. Your proportion would be: _____ cc. : _____ cc. = _____ : _____.

**14**

167 cc.
333 cc.

**14**

When you calculate X, you find that you must use _____ of stock solution and add _____ of diluent to make 500 cc. of finished solution.

**15**

stock solution
diluent

**15**

Let's say that you need to prepare 1/2 gallon of a 1 : 20 solution. The stock solution on hand is 1 : 5 strength.

When you solve for X, you find that the amount of _____ _____ used would be 500 cc. and the amount of _____ added would be 1500 cc.

**16**

400 ml.
600 ml.

**16**

You need to prepare 1 liter of a 1 : 500 solution. The stock solution is labeled 1 : 200; mix _____ of stock solution with _____ of diluent.

**17**

**17**

Up to this point we have worked problems in which the strength of the solution desired and the strength of the solution on hand were both expressed in the same manner, either as a percentage or as a ratio.

There are times, however, when the two strengths are expressed in different terms—one as a percentage and the other as a ratio. In this case we cannot set up a proportion until both strengths are expressed in like terms. Therefore, we must either change the percentage to a ratio or change the ratio to a percentage.

It does not matter which change we make, so long as both strengths are finally expressed in like terms. You already know that it is simple to change a percentage to a ratio: 5% means 5 parts per 100, and can be expressed as the ratio _____ : _____.

5 : 100

**18**

**18**

Let's say that a physician orders an irrigation using a 4% solution. This 4% can be read as the ratio of _____ : 100, or _____ : 1000.

4, 40

**19**

**19**

For practice, change the following percentages to ratios, using as the denominator either 100 or 1000.

(a) 5:100 or 50 : 1000
(b) 1:100 or 10 : 1000
(c) 4.5: 100 or 45 : 1000
(d) 12.5: 100 or 125 : 1000

   (a)   5%
   (b)   1%
   (c)   4.5%
   (d)   12.5%

**20**

**20**

To change a ratio to a percentage, you must first realize that a ratio can be written as a fraction. Once the ratio has

1/10%

been changed to a fraction, it can be changed to percentage by multiplying by 100. Thus the ratio 1 : 1000 becomes the fraction 1/1000, and 1/1000 × 100 = _____ %.

## 21

(a) 8.33%
(b) 25%
(c) 2%
(d) 40%
(e) 1/20 %

### 21

You should be quite proficient in changing ratios to percentages. See if you can work the following problems without difficulty:

(a)  1 : 12   = _____ %
(b)  8 : 32   = _____ %
(c)  1 : 50   = _____ %
(d)  2 : 5    = _____ %
(e)  1 : 2000 = _____ %

## 22

X ml : 3000 ml.
= 1/4000 :
2/100

### 22

Now let's say that you need to prepare 3 liters of a 1 : 4000 solution from a 2% stock solution. If you changed 2% to a fraction, your proportion would be:
X ml.: _____ = _____ : _____.

## 23

X ml. : 3000 ml.
=1/40 %
: 2 %

### 23

If you changed the ratio of 1 : 4000 to a percentage, your proportion would be:
X ml. : _____ = _____ : _____.

## 24

### 24

No matter whether you change the percentage to a ratio or the ratio to a

37.5 ml.

percentage, when you solve for X you will find that you need _____ ml. of the stock solution.

**25**

400 ml.

**25**

Suppose that you need 1/2 gallon of a 1 : 50 solution, and the stock solution on hand is 10%. After setting up your proportion and solving for X, you find that you will need to use _____ of stock solution.

**26**

250 ml.
750 ml.

**26**

If you need to prepare 1000 ml. of a 1% solution, and the stock solution on hand is 1 : 25 strength, you would use _____ of stock solution and _____ of diluent.

**27**

1000 ml.

**27**

A physician orders compresses using a 1 : 20 solution. You will need to prepare 1 gallon of the solution. The stock solution on hand is 20% strength. The amount of stock solution you would use is _____.

**28**

3000 ml.

**28**

Then, to prepare 1 gallon of the finished solution, you would add _____ of diluent to the 1000 ml. of stock solution.

# Post-test on Preparing
# Large Amounts of Solutions

## A. Situations:

1. To prepare 1 gallon of a 4% solution from cresol, which is a pure drug in liquid form, you would use _____ of pure drug and _____ of diluent.

2. To prepare 1000 ml. of a 4% solution from a pure drug in solid form, you would need _____ of pure drug.

3. To prepare 2 gallons of a 1 : 1000 solution from a pure drug in liquid form, you would need _____ of pure drug.

4. To prepare 1 pint of a 0.9% solution from a 10% stock solution, you would use _____ of stock solution in _____ of diluent.

5. To prepare 2 liters of a 1 : 2000 solution from a 2% stock solution, you would need _____ of stock solution and _____ of diluent.

# PART NINE

# PEDIATRIC DOSAGE

**1**

kilograms

**1**

There are available many drug reference books which may be used to find the recommended pediatric dosage, and the average dose is usually given in terms of dosage per kilogram of body weight. If the dosage is given per kilogram of body weight, it may be necessary to convert the weight of the child into _____ .

**2**

kg.

**2**

The abbreviation for kilogram is the first letter of the prefix *kilo*, plus the first letter of the word *gram*. The abbreviation for kilogram is_____.

**3**

2.2 lb. : 1 kg.

**3**

The conversion factor for converting pounds to kilograms is 2.2 lbs. = 1 kg. In converting, the first ratio should be: _____:_____.

**4**

9

**4**

Let's say that an infant weighs 20 pounds. Your proportion is: 2.2 lbs.: 1 kg. = 20 lbs. : X kg. Solving for X, you find that 20 lbs. =_____kg.

**5**

0.09 mg.

**5**

You now know that 20 lbs. is approximately equivalent to 9 kg. If the physician orders atropine, 0.01 mg. per kg. of body weight, the dosage should be _____.

**6**

kilogram

**6**

If you got the correct answer go on to Frame 11. If you are not sure how the answer was obtained, perhaps it would help to review the steps. Your first step is to find out the equivalent of 20 lbs. in kgs., because the dosage is ordered according to _____ of body weight.

**7**

9 kg.

**7**

Use the conversion factor, or 2.2 lbs. = 1 kg. You set up your proportion as 2.2 lbs. : 1 kg. = 20 lbs. : X kg. Solving for X, you find that 20 lbs. is equal to approximately _____ kg.

**8**

0.01 mg.

**8**

The physician has ordered 0.01 mg. per kilogram of body weight. In this next step you use the physician's order as your first ratio. This is written as: _____mg. : 1 kg.

**9**

9 kg.

**9**

The second ratio expresses the unknown dosage in mg. and the 9 kg. which the child weighs. It is written as: X mg. : _____kg.

**10**

0.09 mg.

**10**

Your proportion is:
    0.01 mg. : 1 kg. = X mg. : 9 kg.
Solving for X, you find that the child's dosage should be_____ mg.

**11**

40 kg.

**11**

Suppose the physician orders methylphenidate (Ritalin), 0.75 mg. per kg. of body weight. If the child weighs 88 pounds, his weight in kg. is_____.

**12**

30 mg.

**12**

The dosage ordered is 0.75 mg. per kg. of body weight. The child should receive _____ mg.

**13**

1 1/2 tabs.

**13**

If the medication is available in 20 mg. tablets, you would give the child_____ tablets.

**14**

**14**

The physician orders pyrvinium pamoate (Povan), 5 mg. per kg. of body weight.

16.3 or 16 kg. | The child weighs 36 pounds or_____ kg.

**15**

80 mg. | **15**

The dosage ordered is 5 mg./kg. of body weight. The correct dosage for the child is_____mg.

**16**

8 ml. | **16**

The drug is available in a liquid suspension containing 10 mg. per ml. The child should receive_____ml.

**17**

kilograms | **17**

Suppose you are in a situation in which you feel the need to question a dosage of meperidine hydrochloride (Demerol) which has been prescribed. The dosage ordered is 50 mg. for a child weighing 30 pounds. The recommended dose is 6 mg./kg. of body weight per 24 hours. The first step is to convert the child's weight in pounds into_____.

**18**

13.6 or 14 kg. | **18**

Thirty pounds is approximately equivalent to_____kg.

**19**

**19**

The total amount recommended for a 24-hour period is 6 mg./kg. of body

84 mg.

weight. The total number of mg. allowed in a 24-hour period for this child would be _____ mg.

**20**

14 mg.

**20**

If the drug is given in 6 individual doses, as recommended, each dose should contain no more than _____ mg.

**21**

dangerously
high

**21**

The dosage of 50 mg. of Demerol for a child weighing 30 pounds appears to be · dangerously high/ average/ insufficient ·

**22**

60 mg.

**22**

Mark is a 2-year-old boy just admitted with a diagnosis of acute otitis media. His temperature is 102 degrees Fahrenheit, and he is to receive acetominophen (Tylenol) 5 mg./kg. every 4 hours for a reduction of fever. If Mark weighs 27 pounds, he should receive _____ mg. of Tylenol.

**23**

2.5 ml.

**23**

Tylenol Elixir is available in containers labeled 120 mg./5 ml. You would give Mark _____ ml. every four hours.

**24**

**24**

Mark's orders also include ampicillin trihydrate (Polycillin) 21 mg./kg. of

| | |
|---|---|
| 252 or 250 mg. | body weight every 6 hours. You should give_____mg. of Polycillin every 6 hours. |

| | |
|---|---|
| **25** | **25** |
| 5 ml. | Polycillin is available in a suspension containing 250 mg./5 ml. You would give Mark approximately_____ml. |

| | |
|---|---|
| **26** | **26** |
| 48 | David, age 4, has a diagnosis of bronchial asthma. His orders read 3 mg. Elixophylin per kg. of body weight every 6 hours. If he weighs 36 pounds, you would give_____mg. every 6 hours. |

| | |
|---|---|
| **27** | **27** |
| 9 ml. | Elixophylin is available in an elixir containing 80 mg./15 ml. You can calculate the dosage as_____ml. |

| | |
|---|---|
| **28** | **28** |
| | The use of a drug reference book to determine pediatric dosage eliminates the possibility of error in the calculation of dosage. Whenever the nurse has reason to question a prescribed dosage for a child, it is best to consult such a reference. If, however, a book of this type is not available, one may determine a pediatric dosage by using Clark's rule. |

**29**

adult dosage

**29**

Since many factors must be considered in determining pediatric dosage, Clark's rule is not completely accurate. However, it may be used as a basic guide. The rule is based on two assumptions: First, that the average weight for an adult is 150 pounds, and that the average adult dose is calculated accordingly. The first ratio of weight to adult dosage is 150 lb. : average _____ _____.

**30**

dosage

**30**

The second assumption is that the child's weight in pounds can be compared to the ideal dosage for him in the same way that the average adult weight is compared to the average adult dosage. If the first ratio is 150 lbs. : average adult dose, the second ratio should be child's weight in lbs. : child's _____.

**31**

150

**31**

In Clark's rule then, we are comparing average adult weight to average adult dosage. Since the average adult weight is considered to be 150 lbs., the ratio is _____ lbs. : average adult dose.

**32**

**32**

It is obvious that one must know the average adult dose in order to use Clark's rule. Let's say that the average adult dosage of Aspirin is gr. X. When using Clark's rule, the first ratio would be 150 lbs. : gr. _____.

---

**33**

60

**33**

Continuing with this problem, let's suppose that Mike weighs 60 pounds. The second ratio would be _____ lb. : Mike's dosage.

---

**34**

60 lb. : X gr.

**34**

The proportion would be:

150 lb. : 10 gr. = _____ lb. : _____ gr.

---

**35**

4 gr.

**35**

Solving for X, we find that the dosage of Aspirin for Mike should be _____.

---

**36**

0.1 ml.

**36**

The average adult dosage of Bronkephrine is 0.5 ml. I.M. For an asthmatic attack a child weighing 34 lbs. may receive _____ ml. I.M.

---

**37**

25 mg.

**37**

An adult may be given Benadryl, 50 mg. I.M., for an allergic reaction. A child weighing 75 pounds would receive _____ mg. I.M.

**38**

20 mg.

**38**

The adult dosage for Secobarbital (Seconal) is 100 mg. If a child weighs approximately 30 pounds, the doctor should order approximately_____mg.

**39**

4 cc.,
12.5 mg.

**39**

Mrs. Jackson is to receive 50 mg. of Dramamine for motion sickness. If her daughter, who weighs 37 pounds, has the same illness, it would be most appropriate to give the child · 4 cc. of liquid containing 12.5 mg. / 1/2 of a 50 mg. tablet ·

**40**

adult

**40**

We have said that Clark's rule is based on the assumption that the child's weight in pounds can be compared to the ideal dosage for him in the same way that the average adult weight is compared to the average_____dosage.

**41**

adults

**41**

This assumption can be dangerous owing to the fact that children differ in many ways from _____.

**42**

**42**

Drug companies conduct extensive research studies to determine the ideal child's dosage of each drug. Since each drug is different in its effect on a child, and the circumstances under which a drug may be administered to a child can vary widely, it is strongly recommended that a drug reference book be used to determine the safe and recommended dosage of a specific drug for administra-

child

tion to a _____.

# Post-test on Pediatric Dosage

A. Write the following equivalents:

1. 37 lbs. = _____ kg.
2. 52 lbs. = _____ kg.
3. 16 lbs. = _____ kg.
4. 18 kg. = _____ lb.
5. 42 kg. = _____ lb.

B. Situations:

6. A child is to receive a drug as 2 mg. per kg. of body weight. The child weighs 24 lbs. He should receive _____ mg.
7. A 5-year-old boy is to receive gr. 1/10 per kilogram of body weight. The child weighs 44 lbs. He should receive _____ grains.
8. You may use Clark's rule to determine the pediatric dosage from the average adult dose. The average adult dose is gr. xx. If a child weighs 40 lbs., the pediatric dosage for him is _____ grains.

# PART TEN

# CONVERSION OF FAHRENHEIT AND CELSIUS (CENTIGRADE) TEMPERATURES

**1**

100°C.

**1**

A Celsius thermometer is a centigrade thermometer on which the freezing point of water is 0 (zero) and the normal boiling point of water is 100 degrees (100°C.). The abbreviation for a reading of "one-hundred degrees Celsius" is _____.

**2**

102°F.

**2**

A Fahrenheit thermometer is one on which the freezing point of water is at 32 degrees and the normal boiling point of water is at 212 degrees (212°F.). A reading of "102 degrees Fahrenheit" is abbreviated as _____.

**3**

Fahrenheit

**3**

The Celsius thermometer is becoming increasingly popular as an instrument for measuring body temperature, though the Fahrenheit thermometer may be more familiar to many persons in the health professions as well as to many lay persons. There will be occasions when it may be necessary to convert or "translate" a reading on a Celsius thermometer to a _____ reading which a patient or a member of his family can understand.

**4**

Fahrenheit

**4**

If a child's temperature is found to be 38°C., it may be necessary to explain this number in terms of degrees of temperature on the _____ scale.

**5**

Celsius
 (centigrade)

**5**

There are tables showing Celsius (centigrade) and Fahrenheit equivalents. When such a table is available, one can determine rather quickly the equivalent of a body temperature in either _____ or Fahrenheit.

**6**

proportion

**6**

When a table of equivalents is not readily at hand, it is possible to compute the equivalent using ratio and _____ .

**7**

5°C. :9°F.

**7**

The intervals between 0° and 100° on a Celsius thermometer are evenly divided into units of 5 degrees each. Comparable units on the Fahrenheit scale are equal to 9 degrees each. Using these numbers, we can write the ratio of C. intervals to F. intervals as _____ °C.: _____ °F.

**8**

**8**

Let's say that a temperature of 40°C. is registered on a Celsius thermometer.

40°

You wish to know its equivalent in Fahrenheit degrees. Letting X stand for the unknown number of degrees F., the ratio is written as _____°C. : X°F.

**9**

5°C. : 9°F.

**9**

We have said that the intervals on the Celsius thermometer are given five points each and the intervals on the Fahrenheit thermometer are given 9 points each. Look at the drawing below. The brackets indicate that for every five points on the C. scale there are nine points on the F. scale. The ratio of C. intervals to F. intervals can be written as _____°C. : _____°F.

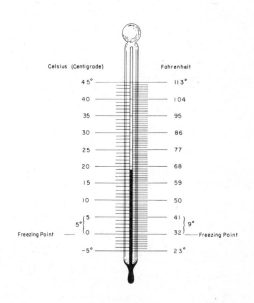

**10**

72°F.

**10**

Now let's get back to the reading of 40°C. for which you wish to know the equivalent in degrees F. The proportion is 40°C. : X°F. = 5°C. : 9°F. Solving for X, you find that X is equal to _____.

**11**

5°

**11**

You have completed the first step in solving the problem of converting degrees C. to degrees F. Now look at the drawing on page 213 again and you will find that a temperature of 41° on the F. scale is equivalent to a temperature of _____ on the C. scale.

**12**

32

**12**

The first interval on the C. scale is given a value of five. The first interval on the F. scale is given a value of 9, which has been added to the number _____, to make a total of 41 degrees.

**13**

F.

**13**

The number 32 is added to the F. reading because the Fahrenheit scale is, so to speak, 32 degrees "ahead of" the C. scale. Since this is the case, we must always add 32 degrees to the Celsius (centigrade) reading when converting from C. to _____.

**14**

32

**14**

As you no doubt have concluded, there are two steps in the conversion of a C. reading to an F. reading.

Step one is to solve for X

Step two is to add _____ to the answer.

**15**

$39°C.:X°F.=$
$5°C. :9°F.$

**15**

Suppose a reading of 39°C. is obtained. The first step in converting this C. reading to an F. reading is to set up a proportion and solve for X. The proportion should be: _____ : _____ = _____ : _____ .

**16**

70.2

**16**

Solving for X, you find that X = _____ .

**17**

32, 102.2°F.

**17**

To the number 70.2, you add _____ to find the Fahrenheit reading of _____ °F.

**18**

add

**18**

You have added 32 to the Celsius reading because the Fahrenheit scale registers 32° at the freezing point, while the Celsius scale registers zero degrees at this point. Whenever you convert from °C. to °F., you must _____ 32 after solving for X.

**19**

97.7°F

**19**

Let's say that you have obtained a reading of 36.5°C. After you set up your proportion and solve for X and add 32, you find that 36.5°C. is equivalent to _____°F.

**20**

100.4°F.

**20**

Suppose you have a reading of 38°C. The equivalent in degrees Fahrenheit is

_____.

**21**

**21**

If you missed the above problem, you may have set up your proportion incorrectly, or you may have failed to add 32 degrees *after* solving for X. It is important that you do not add 32 until after solving for X. Go back to Frame 11 and review the steps for converting degrees C. to degrees F. If you did not miss the problem in Frame 20, continue on to Frame 22.

**22**

32

**22**

There may be an occasion when you will need to convert a Fahrenheit reading to a Celsius reading. The procedure is reversed. The *last* step in converting degrees C. to degrees F. is to *add* 32. The first step in converting degrees F. to degrees C. is to subtract the number

_____.

**23**

98.6

**23**

The number 32 is subtracted from the Fahrenheit reading because the Celsius thermometer registers 0° at the freezing point, while the Fahrenheit thermometer registers 32° at this point. If you have a reading of 98.6°F., and wish to convert to C., your first step is to subtract 32 from _____.

**24**

5°C. : 9°F.

**24**

The answer is 66.6°F. The next step is to set up your proportion:

X°C. : 66.6°F. = _____°C. : _____°F.

**25**

9

**25**

If you missed the above answer, you must have forgotten that the intervals on the Celsius scale are given 5 points each and the intervals on the Fahrenheit scale are given _____ points each.

**26**

5°C. : 9°F.

**26**

The proportion is:

X°C. : 66.6°F. = _____°C. : _____°F.

**27**

37°C.

**27**

Solving for X, you find that X = _____.

**28**

add 32

**28**

For review, let's go over the steps for converting °C. to °F.

Step one: Solve for X

Step two: _____.

**29**

69.3

**29**

For practice, convert a reading of 38.5°C. to a Fahrenheit reading. You set up your proportion and solve for X, finding that X = _____.

**30**

add 32

**30**

To the number obtained for X, you now go to the next step which is to _____ _____.

**31**

101.3°F.

**31**

Your answer of 38.5°C. is equivalent to _____°F.

**32**

107.6°F.

**32**

Now another problem. You have a reading of 42°C. Its equivalent in degrees Fahrenheit is_____.

**33**

subtract 32

**33**

Now let's reverse the procedure. The steps in converting °F. to °C. are:

Step one: _____

Step two: Solve for X.

**34**

39.8°C

**34**

Following these steps you can determine that 103.8°F. is equivalent to a reading of _____°C.

**35**

38.2°C.

**35**

Now try this one. You have a reading of 100.8°F. This is equivalent to _____°C.

**36**

add 32

**36**

The steps for conversion are:

°C. to °F.

Step one: Solve for X

Step two: _____.

subtract 32

°F. to °C.

Step one: _____.

Step two: Solve for X.

# Post-test on Fahrenheit and Celsius Temperatures

Give the equivalents for the following:

1.    35°C.  = _____ °F.
2.    15°C.  = _____ °F.
3.    40°C.  = _____ °F.
4.    86°F.  = _____ °C.
5.  113°F.  = _____ °C.

# Practice Problems

1.  A patient with severe contact dermatitis is to receive cold compresses of Burow's solution (aluminum acetate) in a 1 : 20 dilution 4 times per day. If ℥ xvi of solution are needed for each application, _____ qt(s) will be necessary each day. This is the same as _____ gal.(s).
2.  Mrs. Zolot is receiving 4 ml. of camphorated tincture of opium (paregoric). If each dose is diluted with water to make ℥ i, the nurse will add ℥ _____ of water to the medication.
3.  The medication card reads "Tincture of belladonna ♏ x." If the patient receives this amount 3 times a day, he receives a total of ℥ _____.
4.  The doctor has ordered gr. 1/300. If the drug is available in tablets of gr. 1/150 and gr. 1/600, you would give the patient · two gr. 1/150 tablets/two gr. 1/600 tablets.
5.  Phenprocoumor (Liquamar) is an anticoagulant that is given in varying dosages, adjusted for each individual patient. Let us say that Mr. Good received 21 mg. the first day, 7.5 mg. the second day, 3 mg. the third day, and 0.25 mg. the fourth day. What is the total amount of Liquamar received by Mr. Good in four days? _____.
6.  The initial dose of methylchlothiazide may be as much as 0.01 Gm. daily. If you have this drug available in tablets labeled 5 mg., how many tablets should be given for an initial dose of 0.01 Gm.? _____.
7.  A 3 year old girl is to receive Furoxone 0.033 Gm., 4 times daily. The drug is available in an oral suspension of 16.6 mg./5 ml. How many ml. would the child receive for each dose? _____.

8. A patient with severe myasthenia gravis is to receive Mestinon syrup 0.36 Gm. The dosage on hand is 60 mg./5 ml. How many ml. should he receive? _____ How many ounces is this?_____ .

9. Dimetane is available in elixir labeled 2 mg./5 ml. How much Dimetane is contained in each ml.?_____ .

10. A child who is a clinic patient is to receive 2 teaspoonfuls of Vi-daylin each day. In order to provide a 30-day supply, the patient's mother should receive a · 3 ounce / 8 ounce / pint · bottle to take home.

11. A patient with angina pectoris is receiving nitroglycerin gr. 1/600 as needed for pain. The label on the bottle is 0.1 mg. You should give the patient _____ tablet(s) to provide the dosage of gr. 1/600.

12. The doctor has ordered quinidine sulfate gr. vi. and it is dispensed in tablets of 0.2 Gm. each. You should give _____ tablet(s).

13. A patient is to receive diethylstilbestrol gr. 1/120 and the drug is available in 0.25 mg. tablets. How many tablets should the patient receive?_____ .

14. The doctor has ordered Sodium Nembutal gr. ss intramuscularly. The drug is available in an ampule containing 100 mg./2 ml. You should give the patient _____ minims.

15. A pediatric patient is to receive 0.06 Gm. of Kantrex Pediatric Injection. It is dispensed in vials of 75 mg./2 ml. The patient should receive _____ ml.

16. You have on hand a 4.0 Gm. vial of Staphcillin, and the physician has ordered 1.0 Gm. Directions accompanying the vial read as follows: *Add 5.7 ml. diluent (each 1 ml. contains 500 mg. Staphcillin).* After adding the diluent you should administer _____ ml. to the patient.

17. A physician orders gr. 1/8 and the dosage on hand is a gr. 1/6 hypodermic tablet. To give the patient 15 minims containing gr. 1/8, the nurse should dissolve the gr. 1/6 tablet in _____ minims of diluent and discard _____ minims of solution before giving the injection.

18. A child on the pediatric ward is to receive 3 mg. of Vasoxyl. You have on hand an ampule labeled 10 mg./cc. How many ml. should the child receive? _____. If a tuberculin syringe is not available, how many minims should be given? _____.

19. A pediatric patient is to receive gr. 1/250 of scopolamine as a preoperative medication. The drug on hand is a vial labeled gr. 1/200 per ml. The patient should receive _____ minims.

20. The physician has ordered 6000 units of heparin. The drug is dispensed in an ampule labeled 10,000 units per cc. The patient should receive _____ cc. or _____ minims.

21. Suppose that you were teaching a diabetic patient about insulin. In explaining the difference between U.40 and U.80 insulin, you could say that U.40 was · half as strong/twice as strong · as U.80 insulin.

22. A patient is to receive 60 units of insulin. The drug on hand is U.100 insulin. You should administer _____ ml.

23. In order to prepare one pint of normal saline (0.9%) solution for a throat irrigation, the nurse would need _____ Gm. of pure drug (sodium chloride crystals).

24. To prepare 3 quarts of a 1 : 1000 solution from pure drug in liquid form, you would need _____ ml. of pure drug and _____ ml. of diluent.

25. You must prepare 2 liters of a 1:2000 solution from a 4% stock solution. You will use _____ml. of the stock solution and add _____ ml. of diluent.

# Answers to the Post-test Questions

PART ONE
## INTRODUCTION TO SYSTEMS OF MEASUREMENT

A. Completion

1. system
2. apothecaries', metric
3. household
4. metric
5. apothecaries.'

PART TWO
## THE APOTHECARIES' SYSTEM

A. Table of equivalents

1. 8 drams
2. 16 ounces
3. 2 pints
4. 32 ounces
5. 4 quarts

## B. Abbreviations

6. gal.
7. qt.
8. pt.
9. oz.
10. dr.
11. gr.

## C. Symbols

12. ℥
13. ʒ
14. ℳ

## D. Reading dosages

15. Two and one-half ounces
16. Four ounces
17. Two drams
18. One-half ounce
19. Eight drams
20. Thirteen minims
21. Seven minims
22. Seven and one-half grains
23. Twenty grains
24. Fifteen grains

## E. Charting dosages

25. Mineral oil ʒ iii
26. Cascara ʒ iss.
27. Tincture of belladonna ℳ xv
28. Elixir of Donnatal ʒ ss.
29. Aspirin gr. v

F. Situations

30. 2 quarts    1/2 gallon
31. No.
32. No.
33. 4 5/12 grains
34. 1/64 grain
35. 3 3/4 grains
36. 1/8 grain
37. 1/75 grain
38. 2 tablets
39. 7 1/2 grains

# PART THREE
# THE HOUSEHOLD SYSTEM

A. Situations

1. 1 ounce
2. 1 tablespoonful
3. 1 tablespoonful
4. 2 bottles

# PART FOUR
# THE METRIC SYSTEM

A. Table of equivalents

1. 1000 ml.
2. 1 cc.
3. 1000 mg.

B. Abbreviations

  4. L.                    7. mg.
  5. Gm.                   8. cc.
  6. ml.                   9. mcg.


C. Reading metric abbreviations

  10. Thirty-five hundredths milligram
  11. Two-tenths milligram
  12. One and seventy-five hundredths milligrams
  13. Five-tenths gram
  14. Six-tenths milliliter
  15. Fifty-five hundredths liter
  16. Two and five-tenths milliliters
  17. Four-hundredths milligram
  18. Four and eight-tenths liters
  19. Seven and five-tenths grams
  20. Ten micrograms


D. Charting dosages

  21. 1.5 Gm.
  22. 0.3 mg.
  23. 0.07 ml.
  24. 0.75 L.
  25. 2.5 mg.


E. Situations

  26. 2 bottles
  27. 3 tablets

28. 6 tablets
29. 1 tablet
30. 10 cc.
    0.4 Gm.
31. 5 tablets
32. 2 tablets
33. 8 cc.
    5 days
34. 2 capsules
35. 200 mg.
    1 tablet


PART FIVE
# EXCHANGING UNITS OF WEIGHT AND MEASURE BETWEEN THE APOTHECARIES' AND THE METRIC SYSTEMS

A. Table of equivalents

1. 2 liters
2. 4 liters
3. 2000 ml.
4. 2 pints
5. 30 ml.
6. 2 drams
7. 30 minims
8. 10 minims
9. 1 1/3 ml.
10. 2 ml.
11. 0.02 Gm.
12. 0.5 Gm.
13. 3 3/4 grains
14. 30 grains
15. 3 grains


B. Situations

16. 2 L.
17. 4 ml.
    gr. iiss

18. gr. iii
19. 2 tablets
20. 6 tablets
21. 1 tablet
22. 2 tablets
23. 3 tablets
24. 2 tablets
25. 1/2 tablet

## PART SIX
# PREPARING SOLUTIONS FOR PARENTERAL ADMINISTRATION

A. Situations

1. 1 ml.
2. 0.5 ml.
3. 1.5 ml.
4. 2 tablets
   1.3 ml.
5. 9 minims
6. 1.5 ml.
7. 6 minims
8. 1.5 ml.
9. 0.25 ml.
10. U80

## PART SEVEN
# RATE OF FLOW OF INTRAVENOUS FLUIDS

1.  12.5 or 13
2.  62.5 or 63
3.  26.4 or 26
4.  6.2 or 6
5.  62.5 or 63


## PART EIGHT
# PREPARING LARGE AMOUNTS OF SOLUTIONS

A.  Situations

1.  160 ml. of pure drug; 3840 ml. of diluent
2.  40 Gm. of pure drug
3.  8 ml. of pure drug
4.  45 ml. of stock solution; 455 ml. of diluent
5.  50 ml. of stock solution; 1950 ml. of diluent


## PART NINE
# PEDIATRIC DOSAGE

A.  Equivalents

1.  16.8 or 17 kg.
2.  23.6 or 24 kg.
3.  7.2 or 7 kg.
4.  39.6 or 40 lb.
5.  92.4 or 92 lb.

B. Situations

6. 21.8 or 22 mg.
7. 2 grains
8. 5.3 or 5 grains

# PART TEN
# FAHRENHEIT AND CELSIUS TEMPERATURES

1. $95°F.$
2. $59°F.$
3. $104°F.$
4. $30°C.$
5. $45°C.$

# Answers to the Practice Problems

1. 2 quarts
   1/2 gallon
2. ℥ vii
3. ℥ ss
4. two gr. 1/600 tablets
5. 31.75 mg.
6. 2 tablets
7. 10 ml.
8. 30 ml.
   1 ounce
9. 0.4 mg.
10. 8 ounce
11. 1 tablet
12. 2 tablets
13. 2 tablets
14. 9 minims
15. 1.6 ml.
16. 2 ml.
17. 20 minims of diluent; discard 5 minims
18. 0.3 ml.
    4.5 minims
19. 12 minims
20. 0.6 cc.
    9 minims
21. half as strong

22. 0.6 ml.
23. 4.5 Gm.
24. 3 ml. of pure drug
    2997 ml. of diluent
25. 25 ml. of stock solution
    1975 ml. of diluent

# Final Examination

**Part I   Completion**

Instructions: Write the correct answers in the spaces provided.

A.  Write the correct *abbreviation* for each of the following:
1. ounce _____
6. dram _____
2. liter _____
7. grain _____
3. gram _____
8. cubic centimeter _____
4. milliliter _____
9. microgram _____
5. milligram _____
10. one-half _____

B.  Write the correct *symbol* for each of the following:
11. ounce
12. dram

C.  Write the following dosages as they would be read aloud; for example, *gr. xv* is read 15 grains.
13. ℥ iiss _____
14. ʒ ii _____
15. 0.4 ml. _____
16. 0.25 mg. _____
17. gr. ix _____
18. 0.1 Gm. _____
19. 0.5 L _____
20. 4 mcg. _____
21. 2.5 cc. _____

D. Chart the following dosages using the correct symbols, abbreviations and numbers.
   22. Two ounces _____
   23. One and one-half drams _____
   24. Ten grains _____
   25. Two and one-half grams _____
   26. Four-tenths milligram _____
   27. Three hundredths milliliter _____
   28. One-half liter _____
   29. Three milligrams _____
   30. Eight micrograms _____

E. Complete the following equivalents.
   31. _____ drams = 1 ounce
   32. _____ ounces = 1 pint
   33. _____ pints = 1 quart
   34. _____ ounces = 1 quart
   35. _____ quarts = 1 gallon
   36. _____ liters = 1 quart
   37. _____ milliliters = 1 pint
   38. _____ milliliters = 1 ounce
   39. _____ milliliters = 1 dram
   40. _____ minims = 1 milliliter
   41. _____ grains = 1 gram

F. Write the equivalents:
   42. 98.6°F. = _____ C.
   43. 104°F. = _____ C.
   44. 35°C. = _____ F.
   45. 15°C. = _____ F.
   46. 20 lbs. = _____ kg.
   47. 14 lb. = _____ kg.
   48. 46 lb. = _____ kg.
   49. 28 lb. = _____ kg.

## Part II. Situations

50. The order is to give 0.125 Gm. of an injectable powdered drug. Directions accompanying the drug read *Add 1.7 ml. of diluent (each ml. will contain 500 mg.).* To give the patient 0.125 Gm. of the drug, you would inject the patient with _____ ml.

51. The average adult dosage is gr. xv. The weight of the child is 50 pounds. Using Clark's rule the correct dosage for the child would be _____ .

52. The physician has calculated that the patient should receive 3000 ml. of I.V. fluid every 24 hours by continuous drip. If you are using an I.V. administration set labeled 10 drops per milliliter, the rate of flow will be _____ .

53. A pediatric patient is to receive 500 ml. of fluid I.V. in 6 hours. Using the pediatric I.V. administration set labeled 60 drops per ml., the child will receive _____ drops per minute.

54. You must prepare one gallon of a 1% solution and the stock solution on hand is 1:25 strength. You should use _____ ml. of stock solution and _____ ml. of diluent.

55. Temaril gr. 1/25 is ordered to relieve itching. If the label on the bottle reads 2.5 mg., the patient should receive _____ tablet(s).

56. Another patient on the dermatology unit is receiving Periactin gr. 1/15, four times daily. Grains 1/15 is the same as _____ mg.

## Part III.  Multiple Choice

Instructions:  Choose the one BEST answer. Indicate the answer of your choice by circling the letter preceding it.

57. The physician orders 0.015 Gm. of a certain drug. The drug is dispensed in tablets of 5 mg. each. The patient should be given:
    A.  1/3 tablet
    B.  2 tablets
    C.  3 tablets
    D.  1/2 tablet
58. The physician orders 2 Gm. of a certain medication. The drug is available in 400 mg. tablets. How many tablets should be given to the patient?
    A.  2 tablets
    B.  5 tablets
    C.  4 tablets
    D.  1/2 tablet
59. An elderly patient is to receive 1.25 mg. of a certain drug. He has difficulty swallowing and you have the choice of using a 2.5 mg. tablet or a liquid preparation in which 4 ml. liquid contains 0.625 mg. It would be in the best interest of the patient for you to:
    A.  dissolve the tablet and give him half the solution
    B.  take two tablets to his bedside and encourage him to try to swallow them one at a time.
    C.  give him 8 ml. of the liquid preparation in a small amount of water
    D.  give him 80 ml. of the liquid in an equal amount of water

60. Mrs. Jones is to receive 500 mg. Gantrisin. The only tablets available are 0.25 Gm. each. To supply the dosage as prescribed, you would give her:
   A.   5 tablets
   B.   1/2 tablet
   C.   1 tablet
   D.   2 tablets

61. The doctor has ordered 0.2 Gm. You have available tablets of 50 mg., 100 mg., and 200 mg. each. It would be best to give this patient:
   A.   four tablets of 50 mg. each
   B.   two tablets of 100 mg. each
   C.   two tablets of 50 mg. each
   D.   one tablet of 200 mg.

62. A physician orders gr. ii of a certain drug and the dosage on hand is 60 mg. tablets. You set up your proportion to read:
   A.   60 mg. : 1/2 gr. = 2 gr. : X mg.
   B.   60 mg. : 1 gr. = X mg. : 2 gr.
   C.   30 mg. : 1 gr. = 2 gr. : X mg.
   D.   30 mg. : 1 gr. = X mg. : 2 gr.

63. Suppose a physician orders atropine gr. 1/150, and the label on the bottle reads 0.2 mg. per tablet. You must know how many tablets to give the patient, but first you must convert milligrams to grains.

   After setting up your proportion and calculating X, you find that:
   A.   0.2 mg. = gr. 1/150
   B.   0.4 mg. = gr. 1/150
   C.   0.6 mg. = gr. 1/150
   D.   0.8 mg. = gr. 1/150

64. In another situation, you find that the physician has ordered 3 mg. of a certain drug and that the dosage on hand is tablets of gr. 1/20. In order to give the correct dosage you would use:
A. 1/3 tablet
B. 1/6 tablet
C. 1 tablet
D. 3 tablets

65. The dosage ordered by the physician is gr. 3/4. The drug on hand is in tablets of 15 mg. each. How many tablets should the patient receive?
A. 1/3 tablet
B. 3/4 tablet
C. 1 and 1/3 tablets
D. 3 tablets

66. The physician orders gr. 1/300 (H), and the drug is dispensed in hypodermic tablets of gr. 1/100 each. In order to give the correct dosage, you should dissolve:
A. 1 tablet in 3 ml. of diluent and give 1 ml. of solution
B. 3 tablets in 1 ml. of diluent and give 1 ml. of solution
C. 1 tablet in 1 ml. of diluent and give 1 ml. of solution
D. 3 tablets in 1 ml. of diluent and give 0.5 ml. of solution

67. The physician orders gr. 1/150 (H), and the drug is dispensed in tablets of gr. 1/100 each. In order to give the correct dosage you should dissolve:
A. 1 tablet in 1 ml. of diluent and give 0.5 ml.
B. 1 tablet in 1.5 ml. of diluent and give 1 ml.
C. 2 tablets in 1.5 ml. of diluent and give 0.5 ml.
D. 2 tablets in 2 ml. and give 1.5 ml.

68. Your problem is to give 75 mg. of a drug and you have on hand hypodermic tablets of 30 mg. each. You should use:
    A. 4 tablets, dissolve them in 15 minims and give 10 minims of solution
    B. 4 tablets, dissolve them in 18 minims and give 10 minims of solution
    C. 3 tablets, dissolve them in 15 minims and give 10 minims of solution
    D. 3 tablets, dissolve them in 18 minims and give 15 minims of solution

69. The physician has ordered 6 mg. and the label on the multidose vial reads 25 mg. per ml. You should give the patient:
    A. 0.24 ml.
    B. 0.48 ml.
    C. 2.4 ml.
    D. 4.1 ml.

70. The physician orders Demerol 20 mg. for a child in pediatrics. The label on the vial reads 25 mg. per 0.5 ml. You should give the child:
    A. 0.1 ml.
    B. 0.2 ml.
    C. 0.3 ml.
    D. 0.4 ml.

71. The physician orders 0.4 mg. The drug is available in a multidose vial labeled gr. 1/150 per ml. You should give the patient:
    A. 12 minims
    B. 14 minims
    C. 15 minims
    D. 30 minims

72. The physician orders 3000 units. The drug is dispensed in vials of 5000 units per ml. The patient should receive:
    A.   3 minims
    B.   4.5 minims
    C.   9 minims
    D.   12 minims
73. You are asked to give 15 units of insulin and the drug on hand is U.20 insulin. There is no insulin syringe available. The most accurate dosage would be given if you gave the patient:
    A.   0.75 ml., using a tuberculin syringe
    B.   3/4 ml., using a syringe calibrated in minims
    C.   0.75 ml., using a syringe calibrated in minims
    D.   3/4 ml., using a tuberculin syringe
74. A physician orders 75 units of insulin. An insulin syringe is not available. It would be in the best interest of the patient if you gave:
    A.   14 minims of U.80 insulin
    B.   28 minims of U.40 insulin
    C.   0.75 ml. of U.100 insulin
    D.   1.8 ml. of U.80 insulin
75. A child on pediatrics is given a 2.5 ml. dropperful of medication 4 times a day. If each 2.5 ml. contains 100 mg., the child is receiving a total daily dose of:
    A.   10 ml. containing 0.4 Gm.
    B.   2.5 ml. containing 400 mg.
    C.   5 ml. containing 0.4 Gm.
    D.   10 ml. containing 40 Gm.

# Answers to Final Examination

## Part I. Completion

A. Abbreviations
   1. oz.
   2. L.
   3. Gm.
   4. ml.
   5. mg.
   6. dr.
   7. gr.
   8. cc.
   9. mcg.
   10. ss.

B. Symbols
   11. ℥
   12. ℨ

C. Dosages as Read Aloud
   13. Two and one-half ounces
   14. two drams
   15. four-tenths milliliter
   16. twenty-five hundredths milligram
   17. nine grains
   18. one-tenth gram
   19. one-half liter
   20. four micrograms
   21. two-and-five-tenths cubic centimeters or two-and-one-half cubic centimeters

D. Chart the following dosages:
   22. ℥ ii
   23. ℨ iss
   24. gr. x
   25. 2.5 Gm.
   26. 0.4 mg.
   27. 0.03 ml.
   28. 0.5 L.
   29. 3 mg.
   30. 8 mcg.

E. Equivalents
    31. 8
    32. 16
    33. 2
    34. 32
    35. 4
    36. 1
    37. 500
    38. 30
    39. 4
    40. 15
    41. 15
F. Equivalents
    42. 37°C.
    43. 40°C.
    44. 95°F.
    45. 59°F.

    46. 9 kg.
    47. 6.3 or 6 kg.
    48. 20.9 or 21 kg.
    49. 12.7 or 13 kg.

## Part II. Situations

    50. 0.25 ml.
    51. gr. v
    52. 21 drops/min.
    53. 83 drops/min.
    54. 1000 ml. of stock solution
        3000 ml. of diluent
    55. one tablet
    56. 4 mg.

## Part III.  Multiple Choice

| | | | |
|---|---|---|---|
| 57. | C | 67. | B |
| 58. | B | 68. | D |
| 59. | C | 69. | A |
| 60. | D | 70. | D |
| 61. | D | 71. | C |
| 62. | B | 72. | C |
| 63. | B | 73. | A |
| 64. | C | 74. | C |
| 65. | D | 75. | A |
| 66. | A | | |